DEALING WITH DEMENTIA

DEALING WITH DEMENTIA

A guide to Alzheimer's disease and other dementias

BRIAN DRAPER

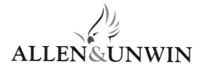

ALLEN&UNWIN

To my family—Debbie, Leah and Sally

First published in Australia by Allen & Unwin in 2004

Copyright © Brian Draper 2004

Allen & Unwin
83 Alexander Street
Crows Nest NSW 2065
Australia
Phone: (61 2) 8425 0100
Fax: (61 2) 9906 2218
Email: info@allenandunwin.com
Web: www.allenandunwin.com

National Library of Australia
Cataloguing-in-Publication entry:

Draper, Brian.
Dealing with dementia: a guide to Alzheimer's disease and other dementias.
Includes index.

ISBN 1 86508 853 6.

1. Dementia. 2. Dementia—Diagnosis. 3. Dementia—Patients—Care. 4. Alzheimer's disease. 5. Alzheimer's disease—Diagnosis. 6. Alzheimer's disease—Patients—Care.
I. Title.

616.83.

Set in 11/13.5 pt Janson by Midland Typesetters, Maryborough, Victoria
Printed by and bound by SRM Production Services, SDN, BHD, Malaysia

10 9 8 7 6 5 4 3 2 1

CONTENTS

LIST OF ILLUSTRATIONS

LIST OF TABLES

PREFACE

Alzheimer's disease is a form of dementia that today is well understood in the community as a major cause of memory impairment and progressive, usually irreversible, mental decline in old age. While many other conditions can cause dementia, Alzheimer's disease is the most common and attracts the greatest attention. Many well-known people, including former US president Ronald Reagan, actor Charlton Heston and author Iris Murdoch (whose illness was portrayed in the movie *Iris*) are openly mentioned as sufferers. Most of us know of someone with the disorder; frequently it is a family member.

Memory impairment in old age has long been recognised as common, but until about 30 years ago was usually regarded as a normal part of the ageing process (senescence). In the 1970s, post-mortem studies of the brains of older people who were senile when they died revealed the microscopic appearances of Alzheimer's disease, which up until that point was believed to be a rare condition afflicting people between 40 and 60 years of age. Named after the German neurologist Alois Alzheimer, who first reported it in 1906, Alzheimer's disease was little more than a footnote in most medical textbooks.

Dramatic changes have taken place since that discovery in the 1970s. Alzheimer's disease, along with other dementias, is now recognised as a major public health concern and has become the target of action plans at all levels of government. There are currently around 165 000 persons with dementia among Australia's 19 million population. The personal and social costs of the disease are enormous.

Largely ignored by medical researchers in the past, Alzheimer's disease is now the focus of numerous public and private research efforts worldwide, with attempts underway to identify causal factors, preventive measures, treatments and even cures. Textbooks, journals and conferences are now devoted entirely to Alzheimer's disease. Alzheimer's Associations and other organisations to support carers of people with dementia have been formed worldwide. In the past five years, drug treatments that offer temporary improvement for some and hope for many have become available. There is even anticipation of a vaccine. Interest in Alzheimer's disease is also burgeoning in the media. This growing awareness has led to increasing numbers of concerned older people presenting to their doctors with mild memory changes which in some cases do represent the earliest symptoms of Alzheimer's disease.

Perhaps you know someone with Alzheimer's disease, are worried about your own memory or are simply curious about the condition. This book is not a medical manual. It is intended to provide an overview of the course of Alzheimer's disease and other dementias, current treatments and the directions being taken by research. I use fictional case studies to illustrate various aspects. I write from an Australian perspective but the principles behind the discussion are widely applicable.

The early chapters set the scene by describing the various causes of memory impairment. In recent years enough has been learnt about the risk factors for Alzheimer's disease and other dementias to allow plausible action to be taken during early to mid adult life that may reduce to varying degrees the risk of developing dementia in old age. The common types of dementia are explained, particularly Alzheimer's disease, vascular dementia, dementia with Lewy bodies and frontotemporal dementia, and how they can be distinguished from each other. An important message is that many other conditions which can affect memory are potentially reversible, including stress, anxiety, depression and the effects of medication, alcohol and other drugs.

The assessment process required to make an accurate diagnosis of dementia is outlined in some detail. While most assessment centres follow the same basic approach, some quite significant individual differences are mentioned. The crucial aspect is the development of a collaborative management plan involving the person with dementia, their family, doctors and other health care personnel.

The treatments available for Alzheimer's disease and some other dementias are covered in Chapters 7 and 8. It is important to understand the indications for, and limitations of, drug treatments for dementia. Some drugs are designed to treat psychological symptoms such as depression, anxiety and hallucinations. Others may improve memory and concentration. The different types of drugs available are covered, along with a range of naturopathic and herbal remedies. Many psychosocial treatments are also used in dementia care, most being designed to improve the quality of life of both the person with dementia and their carers. An overview of these therapies is provided, including validation therapy, reality orientation, aromatherapy and music therapy, to name a few.

Most dementia care is provided by family carers. Without the support of family and friends, it is difficult for the person with dementia to remain in their own home. Initially that support is largely emotional; in the later stages it is also physical. Caregiving can be both rewarding and stressful, often at the same time. Aspects of caregiving, including the important role of the Alzheimer's Association, are the focus of Chapter 9. Formal community support, provided by both government and non-government agencies, has built considerably over the last fifteen years in Australia. A plethora of services devoted to providing practical assistance around the home, respite for the carer and activities for the dementing person has been developed to enable home-based care to be practicable for as long as possible. All such services are based upon the principle of accurate assessment, both of the underlying cause of the mental decline and of the actual needs of the dementing person and their carers. For most lay people the choice can appear bewildering. Chapter 10 outlines, albeit from an Australian perspective, the main types of services available in most developed countries.

There comes a time for most persons with dementia when it is beyond the resources of family and formal community services to maintain them in their home and they must move into residential care. The options include hostels, special care units and nursing homes. Choosing the best option for the individual can be very difficult, and is often limited by availability. Chapter 11 provides some hints to help carers in making the choice. Staff in residential care facilities face many of the same problems encountered by family carers—job satisfaction is mixed with stress and frustration.

There are numerous legal aspects to be considered in dealing with dementia, including assigning power of attorney, guardianship, the dementing person's ability to make a will or even drive a car. Early planning, with the involvement of the dementing person, can often avoid snags later on. When this has not been possible, a formal assessment of mental competency may be required. There are also ethical dilemmas to be faced. What should we do when a dementing person is living alone in squalid conditions and refuses all help? Should we tube feed a person with severe dementia who is unable to swallow safely? These and other common problems are dealt with in Chapter 12.

In the final chapter I have enlisted assistance from dementia specialists from Australia and around the world to ponder the possibilities for early detection, prevention, effective treatment and perhaps cure of Alzheimer's disease and other dementias. The common theme is that we are on the brink of major breakthroughs that will dramatically change the impact of Alzheimer's disease and other dementias. I would like to thank Professor Henry Brodaty from Sydney, Associate Professor David Ames from Melbourne, Professor Colin Masters from Melbourne, Professor Perminder Sachdev from Sydney, Dr Michael Woodward from Melbourne, Professor Brian Lawlor from Dublin, Professor Simon Lovestone from London and Professor Gary Small from Los Angeles for assisting with ideas for this chapter.

I have had a lot of support from my family in writing this book, with my wife Debbie giving very sensible advice on the text, my daughter Sally doing the preliminary sketches for the illustrations in Chapter 5, and my other daughter Leah providing encouragement. The editorial staff at Allen & Unwin, particularly Emma Cotter, Emma Singer and Ian Bowring, have been very helpful in shaping a number of the chapters.

I would like to acknowledge Dr Peter Schofield for permission to reprint Figure 2.1 in Chapter 2, Professor Henry Brodaty for permission to reprint the GP-COG scale in Chapter 6, and Austroads for permission to reprint parts of their advice on fitness to drive for people with dementia in Chapter 12. I would also like to thank Angelo Vlachoulis from the Medical Illustration Unit at Prince of Wales Hospital for the illustrations in Chapter 5.

Brian Draper, 2003

CHAPTER 1

WHAT IS DEMENTIA?

W E LIVE IN AN ageing world. Over the last century life expectancy in Australia has increased from around 55 years to 81.3 years in women and from 52 years to 75.6 years in men.[1] With more people living beyond their allotted 'three-score and ten' years, age-related conditions including osteoarthritis, osteoporosis, cataracts, stroke, cancer, coronary artery disease and dementia have increasingly impacted upon the health of our community. Of these conditions, dementia is the condition that evokes the greatest fear in those contemplating the prospect of a lengthy old age. The possibility of becoming mentally incompetent, forgetful and dependent, in other words senile, can be very disturbing.

DEFINING DEMENTIA

First, let me clarify a few terms. 'Dementia' is a term used medically to describe a *syndrome* (set of symptoms) that is caused by many different diseases. These include Alzheimer's disease, vascular dementia and dementia with Lewy bodies. An analogy is the term 'cancer', which is used to describe any malignant tumour but is not itself a specific disease. The answer to the frequently posed question 'What is the difference between Alzheimer's disease and dementia?' is that, in a sense, there is no difference—Alzheimer's disease is one of the many different types of dementia.

The *dementia syndrome* is defined as an acquired decline in memory and thinking (cognition) due to brain disease that results in significant impairment of personal, social or occupational function. Other brain functions that are affected include orientation,

1

comprehension, calculating ability, learning capacity, language, judgement, reasoning and information processing. While there are some notable exceptions, as I discuss later, dementia is usually of gradual onset and progressive. The World Health Organization (WHO) guidelines recommend that these symptoms and impairments be evident for at least six months before a confident diagnosis can be made.[2] While most dementias are currently irreversible, this does not mean that dementia is untreatable. Its progression (course) can often be influenced and many symptoms can be ameliorated. As I discuss in later chapters, major advances have occurred over the last decade in this area.

Most dementing illnesses are progressive, and early symptoms and problems differ markedly from those in later stages. This may simply be a matter of degree—for example, mild memory impairment moving to profound memory impairment. Other symptoms and problems usually develop later in the course of the illness, urinary incontinence being one example. While it is customary to describe dementia in stages, there is overlap between stages and it may not always be easy to state precisely which stage a person has reached. The first stage is a 'pre-dementia' stage, also named by some researchers 'mild cognitive impairment'. Currently we are unable to identify accurately and reliably what it constitutes. The next three stages, as commonly described to carers during a diagnostic assessment, are 'early' or 'mild', 'moderate' or 'middle' and 'late' or 'severe' dementia, respectively. The final stage, 'advanced dementia', is usually found only in nursing home residents. The stages should be regarded as a guideline rather than as a sacrosanct statement about the person's progress (see Table 1.1).

HOW DOES DEMENTIA DIFFER FROM NORMAL AGEING?

Unlike dementia, the concept of normal ageing is poorly understood. Many of the accompaniments of ageing that result in disabilities in recent times have become treatable, which challenges the notion that they are inevitable features of the physiological ageing process and suggests that they may be considered pathologic conditions. Efforts to characterise mental changes intrinsic to normal ageing are fraught with difficulty, with terms such as 'benign senescent forgetfulness', 'age-associated memory impairment' and 'age-associated cognitive decline' being used and now

Table 1.1 The stages of dementia

Stage	Clinical features
Pre-dementia, questionable dementia, or mild cognitive impairment	There is no set pattern; the various symptoms may occur independently of each other and are often only recognised retrospectively: • Subjective awareness of short-term memory deficits and/or close friends/relatives notice a mild change • Depression and anxiety along with other non-specific behaviour or memory changes • Personality changes such as apathy and irritability often attributed to age or depression • Close relationships might become strained, less social and hobby activities • Work performance, decision-making and problem-solving difficulties may occur
Mild or early dementia	Consistent deficits across a range of domains, however usually still able to function with minimal assistance: • Impairment in short-term memory interferes with day-to-day function, e.g. losing keys, forgetting conversations • Some disorientation in time, e.g. date, and may become disorientated when in unfamiliar places • Some word-finding difficulties—names, objects • Obvious difficulties with problem solving, especially in novel situations • Difficulties in social functioning, e.g. shopping, finances or business affairs, though may superficially appear normal and engage in them • More difficult household tasks no longer done and less interest in hobbies • May require prompting in personal care

continues . . .

Table 1.1 The stages of dementia (continued)

Stage	Clinical features
Moderate or middle stage dementia	More severe deficits, clearly needs assistance from a carer to function at a level comparable to before onset of dementia: • Severe memory loss and rapidly forgets new information • Usually disoriented in time and often as to place • Obvious difficulties in finding words, often doesn't speak spontaneously • Starts to misidentify familiar people • Problem solving and judgement very poor • Unable to function independently in social situations, but is usually able to attend with supervision • Only able to perform simple chores at home • Requires assistance with personal care • Behavioural difficulties emerge, e.g. wandering, agitation, aggression, psychosis, sleep disturbance
Severe or late stage dementia	No semblance of independent function; the majority of persons with severe dementia are in residential care: • Very severe memory loss, only fragments remain • Oriented to person only • Unable to solve problems or make judgements • Language skills limited to a few words and phrases • Regularly misidentifies familiar people • Social function is minimal even with supervision • No significant self-care capacity • Frequent incontinence • Behavioural difficulties increase

Table 1.1 The stages of dementia (continued)

Stage	Clinical features
Advanced dementia	Completely dependent on carers for all aspects of daily living: • No semblance of memory function • Usually inarticulate, may be mute • Cannot identify familiar people • Very poor comprehension of simple verbal commands • Social interactions virtually non-existent • May lose capacity to stand, walk and sit up • Incontinent of urine and faeces

generally reflect the extremes of normal ageing rather than describing a precursor of pathologic ageing.

We acquire knowledge through an active cognitive processing of information that involves thinking, learning and remembering; it is known as fluid intelligence. Fluid intelligence tends to decline with age. Short-term memory wanes to a degree, but in contrast to a person with dementia who tends to forget a whole experience the normal older person will only forget parts of the experience. For example, where the person with dementia might forget altogether having been to the cinema, the normal older person might just forget some details of the film. New learning becomes more difficult for the normal older person, the ability to solve novel problems declines and the speed of mental processing slows. There is a speed–accuracy trade-off, however, with the normal older person tending to make fewer errors.

There is also an age-related tendency to have some increased difficulty in word-finding and remembering names—a situation that most of us have experienced as having a word 'on the tip of the tongue'. In most cases the missing word appears a bit later without prompting. Associated anxiety about not getting the word out may often magnify the problem. In addition, those people who are more 'tongue-tied' than others and have always had some difficulties in expressing themselves find that the ageing process exacerbates this tendency.

The accumulation as one ages of all the knowledge and products of previous cognitive processes is known as 'crystallised intelligence'. Crystallised intelligence does not decline in normal ageing; rather, it often increases with maturity and brings greater wisdom. It is one of the reasons that societal elders are held in high regard and hold senior positions in most cultures.[3]

There is no precise point at which normal age-related cognitive changes can be said to become a pathological entity (disease), and there is considerable debate on the issue in the scientific community. There are, however, some warning signs. Normal age-related decline takes place over decades, so decline over a shorter time, months or a few years, is liable to be pathological. This is particularly the case if the person's functional performance has declined relative to their peers and they are unable to adapt to maintain functioning in normal life.

WHAT ARE THE MAIN TYPES OF DEMENTIA?

Alzheimer's disease is the most common type of dementia in most countries in the world, the main exceptions being Japan and China where vascular dementia predominates. Alzheimer's disease accounts for about 50 to 60 per cent of dementia cases, sometimes occurring in combination with other dementias. Vascular dementia is the next most common, accounting for 15 to 20 per cent of cases. Mixed Alzheimer's-vascular dementia is probably more widespread than clinical diagnoses would suggest, with some post-mortem studies suggesting that it might involve as much as 25 per cent of dementia cases. Over the past decade, dementia with Lewy bodies has become increasingly recognised and is said to account for up to 20 per cent of cases, though it would seem that many of these cases also have Alzheimer's disease.[4] Frontotemporal dementia, which includes Pick's disease, occurs in approximately 10 per cent of cases and is particularly common in younger age groups.

Numerous other conditions can cause dementia, but most of them are rare. Conditions such as alcohol abuse, hypothyroidism, vitamin B_{12} deficiency and Parkinson's disease are regularly found in persons with dementia, but in most cases the main cause is Alzheimer's disease or vascular dementia. Well-known rare causes of dementia include brain tumours, normal pressure hydro-cephalus, progressive supranuclear palsy, cerebral vasculitis and brain trauma. In younger age groups, Human Immunodeficiency Virus (HIV)-related disorders are a more prominent cause, though it should be stressed that in most cases other HIV-related disorders have been previously diagnosed and the dementia occurs late in the course of the disease.

HOW COMMON IS DEMENTIA?

To date over 100 studies worldwide have reported on the prevalence of dementia. Most have been undertaken in developed countries. Professor Tony Jorm and colleagues from the Australian National University in Canberra pooled data from 22 studies and found that the prevalence of dementia doubled every 5.1 years from the age of 60. Applying these rates to the estimated Australian population in 2000 would translate to the figures in Table 1.2, with an overall prevalence of approximately 155 500 persons,[5] revealing that dementia is an age-related condition and its occurrence under the age of 60 is quite rare. While there have been no Australian studies, research from the United States suggests that there are likely to be only around 1300 persons with dementia in the 50–59 age group in Australia, and a further 1000 under the age of 50.

Table 1.2 Estimated prevalence of dementia in Australia in 2000, persons aged 45 years and over

Age group	Prevalence rate (%)	Estimated population (1000s)	Estimated prevalence of dementia
45–49	0.077	1342.6	1 034
50–54	0.04	1245.0	498
55–59	0.086	958.4	824
60–64	0.7	780.8	5 500
65–69	1.4	676.4	9 470
70–74	2.8	625.4	17 511
75–79	5.6	504.2	28 235
80–84	11.1	304.5	33 800
85+	23.6	248.6	58 670
Total		**6685.9**	**155 542**

IS DEMENTIA BECOMING MORE COMMON?

The simple answer to this question is 'yes', but the increase is basically due to the ageing of the population, not to any innate changes in the risk of developing dementia. As more people survive or avoid early and mid-life illnesses such as cardiac and infectious diseases, they live to an age where they are at higher risk of dementia. This is accentuated by the increasing numbers of persons aged over 85 years—the age group at greatest risk.

There is no evidence from the recent past, in studies from Sweden or the USA, to suggest any significant change in the risk of developing dementia at any particular age. In other words, the incidence (the number of new cases developing in a defined time period) of dementia is only increasing due to these population changes. Thus a person aged 70 in 2003 appears to have a similar risk of developing dementia as a person aged 70 had in 1983. What is not known is whether there have been any changes compared with a hundred or more years ago, and whether the incidence will change in 20 years or more remains to be seen. The impact on rates of dementia of altering various lifestyle risk factors, as described in Chapters 2 and 3, is also unknown. Statistically, if it were possible to simply delay the onset of dementia by a year or two, its prevalence would drop by tens of thousands.

One factor that may impact upon the prevalence of dementia is the recent introduction of cholinesterase-inhibitor drugs such as Aricept, Reminyl and Exelon (see Chapter 7) now being pre-scribed for Alzheimer's disease. While their long-term effects are unknown, these agents appear to slow the progress of the disease for around twelve to eighteen months in approximately 50–60 per cent of patients. It has been hypothesised that dementia symptoms will initially be reduced but that eventually, as the disease pro-gresses, there will be a more rapid decline, with death occurring at the same age as without treatment. Most authorities believe that the actual duration of the disease is not likely to be altered by the use of these drugs. But what if it is altered? If the course of the disease is prolonged, the prevalence of dementia will increase simply because more people are surviving with the illness. Thus, the duration of Alzheimer's disease being increased by one year would have a similar but opposite effect to delaying its onset. In other words, the prevalence of dementia cases might *increase* by some tens of thousands! The only published information to date involves the first-released cholinesterase inhibitor, tacrine, which is now rarely used. Contrary to expectations, it has been shown to reduce mortality in advanced dementia. Before too much is made of this finding, other studies are needed, particularly of the newer agents that now dominate the market. It will be some years before it is known whether these agents have any measurable impact upon disease duration.

Without taking the possible impact of cholinesterase-inhibitor drugs and moderation of known risk factors into account, Tony Jorm and colleagues have estimated the increase in the number of dementia cases in Australia in the period 1995 to 2041. While the total Australian population is projected to increase by 40 per cent, from just over 18 million in 1995 to just over 25 million in 2041, the number of persons aged 65 years and over is projected to increase by 166 per cent, from around 2.15 million in 1995 to 5.72 million in 2041. Dementia cases, however, are projected to increase by 254 per cent, from around 130 000 in 1995 to 459 000 in 2041. This marked increase is mainly attributable to the projected increase in the number of persons surviving to age 80 and beyond.[6]

Such projections are not unique to Australia. Other developed migrant countries such as Canada, the United States and New Zealand will see a similar pattern. Old World European countries with stable populations such as Sweden and the United Kingdom will have less dramatic changes, although the prevalence of dementia will still increase. It is in the developing world where the most dramatic changes will take place. Indonesia, for example, is projected to have a 295 per cent increase in dementia cases between 1990 and 2030. China, India and Latin America will also have particularly marked increases.[7]

WHAT IS THE IMPACT OF DEMENTIA UPON SOCIETY?

The global impact of dementia is growing. According to the WHO *World Health Report 2001*, dementia was ranked as the thirteenth leading cause in the world of years lived with a disability in 2000. This ranked ahead of such disorders as cerebrovascular disease, HIV/AIDS, diabetes mellitus and cataracts. It was projected that dementia would rapidly increase its contribution to the global burden of disease over the next 20 years, particularly in developed countries.[8]

These global impacts are mirrored in Australia. The *Australian Burden of Disease and Injury Study*, undertaken by the Australian Institute of Health and Welfare in 1998/99, provides a comprehensive assessment of the amount of ill health and disability, the 'burden of disease', in Australia in 1996. In this study, mortality, disability, impairment, illness and injury arising from 176 diseases, injuries and risk factors were measured using a common tool, the Disability-Adjusted Life Year (DALY). One DALY is a lost year of 'healthy' life. It is calculated from the combination of years of life lost to premature mortality and equivalent 'healthy' years of life lost due to disability.

In 1996 in Australia, dementia was the sixth-ranked leading cause of burden of disease in all ages, accounting for 3.5 per cent of total DALYs. It was ranked fourth in women and tenth in men. Ischaemic heart disease and stroke were the two leading causes of disease burden. In older Australians, dementia ranked third in women and fifth in men. Dementia is the second leading cause of 'healthy' years lost to disability in both men and women of all ages, trailing only depression, which it will overtake by 2016. Dementia was also the sixth leading cause of mortality, and was noted to have one of the largest increases in mortality burden in the period 1981–96. This coincides with the increased recognition and more accurate diagnosis of dementia in Australia, rendering it more likely for doctors to include the diagnosis on death certificates.[9] In 2002, it was estimated that dementia cost over 117 000 years of healthy life.[10]

In March 2003, Access Economics released a report prepared for Alzheimer's Australia on the economic impact of Alzheimer's disease in Australia. The report estimated that there were 162 000 people with dementia in Australia in 2002, 6 600 under 65 years old. The total annual estimated costs of dementia were A$6.6 billion; direct health costs were A$3.2 billion, of which A$2.9 billion was spent on residential care. Access Economics estimated that these costs would double by 2010. Real indirect costs were A$2.4 billion, being costs to carers (A$1.7 billion), lost earnings and the mortality burden of dementia sufferers (A$364 million) and the costs of aids and home modifications

(A$120 million). There was an additional A$1 billion in transfer costs—foregone taxes, carer payments and other welfare payments.[11]

In the USA a number of estimates have been made of the annual costs of caring for a person with dementia. The costs increase with the severity of dementia, being estimated at approximately A$94 000 for a patient with severe dementia. The total direct and indirect costs of caring for dementia in the USA have been estimated as approximately A$180–200 billion per year.[12]

Dementia already has a considerable effect upon the Australian community. The projected massive increase in the number of cases over the next 40 years is likely to further elevate dementia in the list of leading causes of disease burden, though current and future therapies may ameliorate the impact to some degree. In Victoria, dementia has been projected to become the leading cause of disease burden in women and the fifth highest in men by 2016.[13] Such striking increases obviously will have enormous economic consequences, just in meeting the need for more medical, community and residential services to maintain current standards. The dilemma of how to fund such demands from the public purse has been a concern of economists, health care planners and politicians for some time. The move towards self-funded retirement and user-pays principles in provision of services has largely evolved from these projections.

SUMMARY

The dementia syndrome is an acquired decline in memory and thinking processes due to brain disease that results in significant impairment of personal, social and occupational functions. It is not due to a normal ageing process. The most common type of dementia is Alzheimer's disease, though other common types include vascular dementia, dementia with Lewy bodies and frontotemporal dementia. Dementia is increasing in prevalence due to the ageing of the population, and is projected to have a commensurate increase in the economic impact and burden of disease on society.

CHAPTER 2

PREVENTION OF DEMENTIA I

'HOW CAN I STOP myself getting dementia?' is a question commonly posed to dementia specialists. Until recently, it has not been possible to provide any advice based on reputable research. The situation is rapidly changing, however, and in this and the next chapter I describe the known risk factors for dementia and strategies that may possibly counteract them. One of the features of recent research has been the convergence of identified risk factors for the two most common types of dementia, Alzheimer's disease and vascular dementia. Thus I discuss prevention strategies for dementia as a whole and indicate where particular strategies may be important for specific types of dementia.

DISEASE PREVENTION

It is important to appreciate that intentional efforts to prevent any disease imply that there is some reasonable understanding of what causes it. The disease process by which the causal factors turn a normal state into a pathological (diseased) state must also be understood. Recognition of 'risk factors' that may facilitate or are associated with the disease process, and 'protective factors' that may suppress the process or are associated with normality, is also crucial. Risk and protective factors may include genetic, medical, biological, environmental, dietary, social and cultural aspects. In the field of dementia, it has only been over the last decade that knowledge has grown sufficiently in these domains for prevention strategies to be mounted.

Historically, of course, many conditions have been prevented unintentionally or by unknown methods. An example is suicide in

Australian men aged between 45 and 75 years, where annual rates have dropped over the last 40 years from around 38 per 100 000 men to 24 per 100 000. No specific suicide prevention strategies were responsible for the change. While it has been hypothesised that the change might be related to improvements in the general health of men in this age group, no one knows for sure what has been responsible, particularly as suicide rates in younger men have increased dramatically during the same period, and those in men aged over 75 years remain very high.

Disease prevention may involve either elimination or postponement of the disease.

Disease elimination

Disease elimination suits diseases with single known causes (pathogens) that can be specifically targeted in a prevention strategy. This has been the model used in infectious diseases such as smallpox, which was eliminated from the community by population vaccination programs, and in other diseases such as measles, rubella, polio and diphtheria, which can be prevented in most individuals by vaccination. This will also be the model used in proposed gene therapies for genetic disorders where a single gene mutation is responsible for the disease. The gene therapy will target the mutation and correct the abnormality before it has had the opportunity to cause irreparable damage. Another method of disease elimination involves DNA testing of a foetus during early pregnancy where a known genetic risk for a disorder, such as Down syndrome, exists leading to a possible termination of the pregnancy.

As most cases of dementia are likely to be multifactorial in origin, disease elimination is not a realistic objective unless the prevention strategy targets a 'final common pathway' of the disease process. Hopes were raised in 1999 by the publication in the prestigious journal *Nature* of reports of immunotherapy treatment that eliminated beta-amyloid plaques, the major pathological abnormality in the brain in Alzheimer's disease (see Chapter 5). The therapy stimulated the immune system of mice to identify and assault the amyloid plaques. As Alzheimer's disease does not naturally occur in mice, the research involved the transplantation of a rare human Alzheimer's disease gene into the mouse. Immunisation of young transplanted mice with a protein named AN-1792 prevented the development of the beta-amyloid plaques, while immunisation of older mice after they had already developed beta-amyloid plaques halted the further accumulation of beta-amyloid protein and in some cases reversed the process. Later independent studies showed that AN-1792 also improved the performance of these mice on tests designed to measure rodent memory. Once these results hit the media, AN-1792 was quickly dubbed the Alzheimer 'vaccine' (although this is an inaccurate description, 'immunotherapy' being a better term).

These exciting findings quickly led to human trials of AN-1792 with the approval of both the US Food and Drug Administration (FDA) and the UK Medicines Control Agency. Initial trials in 2000 to test its safety in humans (known as Phase I trials) revealed no problems and led to the commencement in 2001 of a small Phase IIA trial in Europe and the United States to begin assessing the drug's effectiveness, to determine the best dosage and to further test safety. The trial enrolled 360 people with mild to moderate Alzheimer's disease. In January 2002, the sponsors, Elan and Wyeth-Ayerst Laboratories, announced suspension of the dosing schedule after four participants who had received multiple doses of AN-1792 developed symptoms of inflammation of the central nervous system. By the end of February 2002, the number of affected participants had increased to fifteen, with several deaths, and the trial was discontinued in March 2002.

Even if these concerns about the safety of AN-1792 are resolved, there are other concerns. A hypothetical concern is the possibility that in provoking an immune reaction to one of the body's own proteins AN-1792 could stimulate an autoimmune reaction in which the body mobilises an indiscriminate onslaught on its own tissues. Also, more recent studies in mice have found an increased risk of cerebral haemorrhage (stroke) in vaccinated mice. Apart from safety, possibly the most important question is whether dissolution of amyloid plaques will actually result in improvement of mental function. Many Alzheimer's experts have expressed doubts about this. There is even doubt about the capacity of AN-1792 to generate a strong enough immune response in humans to have a therapeutic effect. The participants are still being followed up, and in October 2002 it was reported that those who received the vaccine did develop antibodies to beta-amyloid and that there did not appear to be any correlation between an individual's antibody levels and the risk of developing brain inflammation. There is not yet any indication of any effects on trial participants' memory or thinking abilities.[1] In March 2003, the autopsy findings of one of the AN-1792 subjects were reported in *Nature*. They indicated a very large reduction of beta-amyloid plaques in the brain, the desired outome.[2]

So, while there are tantalising suggestions that immunotherapy might provide a therapeutic opportunity to eliminate Alzheimer's disease, it is clearly not going to happen just yet. I explore this theme further in Chapter 13.

Disease postponement

In complex or chronic diseases associated with ageing, such as dementia, disease postponement may be an adequate prevention measure for the foreseeable future. While postponement does not prevent disease, the period of time involved may still have a dramatic effect. Delaying the onset of dementia could allow a person to enjoy a longer period of healthy life, before succumbing to some other condition perhaps before dementia developed, or when their dementia was still relatively mild. In the United States, it has been estimated that if the onset of Alzheimer's disease were delayed by two years, the prevalence of around 2.9 million cases in 2007 would be reduced by around 600 000! Disease postponement is largely about modifying known risk factors of dementia.[3]

PUBLIC HEALTH MODEL OF PREVENTION

The public health model of prevention identifies three types of strategy to prevent disease. *Universal strategies* apply to the whole population, *selective strategies* to individuals at high risk and *indicated strategies* to individuals with early symptoms or indications of disease. These different types of strategy can be applied to dementia prevention. The rest of this chapter outlines some universal strategies; the next chapter covers selective and indicated strategies of dementia prevention.

UNIVERSAL DEMENTIA PREVENTION STRATEGIES

Universal strategies for disease prevention are applied to everybody in a population because all the population is at potential risk of harm from the targeted risk factor. Common examples include water purification to eliminate waterborne infectious diseases in the water supply, hand washing before food handling to prevent bacterial food contamination and treatment of sewage before disposal to prevent bacterial contamination of waterways. Although universal strategies may seem to have only a limited effect for the individual, when applied across a whole population the effect is magnified considerably. A number of dementia risk factors apply to the whole population, so universal strategies are applicable.

AGE AND THE ROLE OF ANTIOXIDANTS

Increasing age is the most established risk factor for dementia, though there is still debate about whether the risk continues to increase after the age of 90. Some authorities believe that there may be a reduction of the risk; others suggest that the rate of dementia in centenarians may be at least 70 per cent. It also remains unclear whether the increased rates of dementia in old age are caused by the ageing process itself or by other diseases or events that are themselves age-related. Obviously we do not want to prevent a person from getting older, but a better understanding of the ageing process and of factors that enhance its effects may lead to some useful prevention strategies.[4]

One particular strategy involving the ingestion of antioxidants may already be informally in place. Antioxidants potentially have a role in preventing dementia. As the brain ages, its capacity to remove certain harmful small molecules known as 'free radicals' is reduced, resulting in cell death and increased susceptibility of nerve cells to other factors that cause damage. The brain cells' natural defences against this damage include manufacturing antioxidants that mop up free radicals, but with age some of these protective mechanisms decline.

Curcumin (from the herb turmeric), alpha-lipoic acid, flavonoids, vitamin B_6, vitamin C, vitamin E and vitamin A are just a few of the many antioxidants available on the shelves in health food stores. A number of these substances have been examined for their ability to prevent Alzheimer's disease, vascular dementia or cognitive impairment, but the results so far are equivocal.

Vitamins C and E

There is modest evidence that vitamins C and E may have a protective role against dementia. The Honolulu–Asia Aging Study found that older men who took supplements of vitamins C and E had lower rates of vascular dementia and cognitive impairment but not Alzheimer's disease. An epidemiological study published in the influential *Journal of the American Medical Association* (*JAMA*) in June 2002 suggested that eating foods rich in antioxidants (such as fibres, grains, fish, green vegetables), especially vitamin E (but not vitamin E supplements), may help lower the risk of developing Alzheimer's disease.[5] A second study published in the *Archives of Neurology* in July 2002 found vitamin E to be protective against memory decline.[6]

An editorial in *JAMA* concluded that while the studies were not conclusive as to whether antioxidant vitamins are truly protective against Alzheimer's disease (because of weaknesses in their design), they supported the view that dietary antioxidant vitamins may prevent the development of Alzheimer's disease.[7] The optimal dose of vitamin E is not known. Many doctors recommend 500 international units (IU) twice daily; this level is safe for most individuals and should have the antioxidant effect desired in the brain. However, people taking anticoagulants such as warfarin may not be able to take vitamin E, and should be monitored closely by their doctor.

At least five clinical trials are currently underway specifically to examine the role of vitamins C and E and other antioxidants in preventing memory decline and Alzheimer's disease; until the results of these trials are available, it is unknown whether vitamin supplements will prevent Alzheimer's disease.

Alcohol (red wine)

It is well established that excessive alcohol intake, usually in combination with thiamine deficiency, can cause brain damage. One well-known type of brain damage is the Wernicke-Korsakoff syndrome, in which profound short-term memory impairment occurs. Unlike dementia, this is not a progressive condition but it is irreversible, leaving the sufferer severely impaired even when alcohol consumption ceases. More controversially, alcohol has long been regarded as a cause of dementia, although precise brain pathology has not been established.

Epidemiological studies have not demonstrated that alcohol is a risk factor for dementia. Indeed, as demonstrated in the Rotterdam Study, light to moderate drinking (one to three drinks per day) was significantly associated with a *lower* risk of any dementia, and vascular dementia in particular, in individuals aged 55 years or older. The effect seemed to be unchanged by the source of alcohol.[8] However, some studies have suggested that red wine may have particular benefit. The flavonoids in wine— powerful antioxidant substances also contained in tea, fruits and vegetables—have been thought to offer protection. One study has found that the intake of antioxidant flavonoids was inversely related to the risk of dementia.[9] While these findings may give some encouragement to drink alcohol in old age, a few words of caution are required. For some individuals there may be a fine line between a potentially beneficial amount of alcohol and a deleterious amount. Further, women experience the deleterious effects of alcohol at much lower amounts than men. Until prospective controlled studies of light to moderate alcohol intake are undertaken, it remains an unproven preventive strategy. In those who have established dementia, relatively small amounts of alcohol can cause increased confusion and behavioural changes.

The lack of strong evidence for the effectiveness of antioxidants in the prevention of dementia should not be viewed too negatively. The lack of evidence does not mean that they are ineffective—it is just that to determine whether a particular antioxidant may be effective requires very large, randomised, placebo-controlled studies, such as the trials underway in the United States involving thousands of subjects monitored over many years.

EDUCATION, INTELLIGENCE AND BRAIN RESERVE

Low levels of formal education have been found to be associated with higher levels of cognitive impairment, dementia in general and Alzheimer's disease in particular. Another way of looking at it is that people with higher levels of education are less likely to develop dementia. In one Canadian study, people with more than ten years of education were four and a half times *less* likely to have dementia than those with less than six years of education. Pooled data from European studies, however, has suggested that the effects of education may only occur in women.[10]

The mechanism of this relationship between education and dementia is unclear but there are a number of possibilities. One possibility is that a low level of education may be a proxy for dele-terious environmental influences. Another is that a high level of education may be a proxy for intelligence, as more intelligent people are likely to obtain more formal education. The evidence that low intelligence may be linked with the development of dementia is quite varied. Lower premorbid intelligence has been found to predict the development of dementia in elderly people. More generally, lower premorbid intelligence predicts a worse cognitive outcome following head injury. Possibly the most intriguing evidence, however, is the Nun Study, in which a cohort of elderly Roman Catholic nuns were assessed, with a number having their brains studied post-mortem. Diary entries written in their late teenage years were examined for linguistic ability. Low linguistic ability during the teenage years was associated with Alzheimer's disease brain pathology at autopsy. One interpreta-tion of these findings has been that incipient Alzheimer's disease was already present in the teenage nuns; certainly, it has been shown that the pathological changes of Alzheimer's disease may be present for 30 to 50 years before its clinical onset. Another interpretation is that the linguistic ability was a proxy for intelligence.[11]

So how might intelligence reduce the risk of dementia? One hypothesis, proposed by Peter Schofield from the University of Newcastle, Australia, is that more intelligent people have a larger 'brain reserve'. The concept of brain reserve is based on the fact that our brains carry redundant neurons that act as a type of back-up in times of need. In this hypothesis, when the brain is damaged, for example by a stroke or through the gradual devel-opment of Alzheimer's disease, the brain reserve comes into play to replace or cover for the damaged cells. If the brain reserve is inadequate to cover for the damage, the threshold of the disease is reached and the person becomes symptomatic. Thus the larger the brain reserve, the greater the damage that can be sustained before symptoms occur. Whether this effect is due to there being 'further to fall' before reaching disease threshold, or whether the large brain reserve in some way resists the neuropathological changes, for example through greater cognitive flexibility, is unclear. Whatever the model, a person with a large brain reserve may have incipient Alzheimer's disease for many years and be asymptomatic (see Figure 2.1). In this situation, intelligence is delaying the onset of dementia.[12]

Other important factors contribute to brain reserve. Any physical damage to the brain may reduce the reserve. This ties in with the finding that head injuries causing loss of consciousness for at least fifteen minutes may increase the risk of Alzheimer's disease up to twofold, though the studies are inconsistent and possibly the most methodologically sound prospective study had a negative result. Boxers may develop 'dementia pugilistica' due to repeated blows to the head and recently Jeff Astle, a former England soccer international, was found to have died from a degenerative brain disease caused by 'heading' the soccer ball,

Figure 2.1 Brain reserve: Two models (Schofield, 1999)

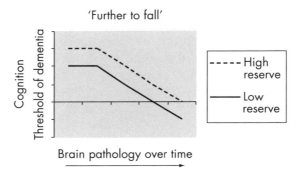

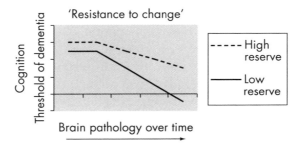

a skill for which he was famous. Other types of previous brain damage, including strokes, and mental retardation may also increase the likelihood of dementia occurring.

Brain size is another factor—the larger the brain, the larger the brain reserve. This may be linked with intelligence, as more intelligent people tend to have larger brains. People with larger brains, as measured by CT scans, MRI scans or head circumference, are less likely to develop the symptoms of Alzheimer's disease, even if they have the features of the disease in their brains at autopsy.

Mental activity also influences brain reserve. It is possible that mental activity enhances neuronal integrity through the action of better cerebral blood flow in reducing levels of stress and improving DNA repair. More tantalisingly, it may also enhance brain growth. A number of studies have shown that engaging in various forms of intellectual activity through life, even in the sixth and seventh decades, may protect against cognitive decline and enhance memory function. In a study published in *JAMA* in 2002, investigators from Rush Presbyterian St Luke's Medical Centre in Chicago followed 801 older Catholic nuns, priests and brothers for almost five years, tracking their everyday activities: reading the newspaper, listening to the radio, playing games such as chess, or watching television. They found that those clergy who did three or more of these things at least several times a week were almost 50 per cent less likely to develop Alzheimer's disease than those who read, listened to the radio and played games only a few times a month.[13]

It may not just be the quantity of mental activity that is important. Deciding to stimulate your brain through a series of repetitive, boring mental exercises, or putting pressure on yourself by taking on an intellectual pursuit that is well beyond your capacity, may both be detrimental. Authors of memory books often recommend mental exercises that include 'pegging' numbers to words for easier recall, visualising pictures with numbers and words, crossword puzzles, logic and graph puzzles, and exercises to improve the recall of word lists. Unless you enjoy doing these things they are unlikely to be of much benefit. Put simply, the mental activity should be fun!

The implications of these findings are that early life events may influence the development of dementia and that participating in varied mental and physical activities through life may impart a protective role.

CEREBRAL BLOOD FLOW

The Chinese herb *Ginkgo biloba* is thought to increase circulation to the brain. In Europe and some Asian countries, standardised extracts from ginkgo leaves are taken to treat a wide range of symptoms, including dizziness, inflammation and reduced blood flow to the brain and other areas of impaired circulation. It is routinely prescribed in Europe for memory problems and although there is some evidence that it may be beneficial, the studies are not strong. The US National Institute on Aging helped fund a trial in which 2000 older adults at risk of dementia took daily doses of ginkgo or a placebo; the results, released in August 2002, were negative. One of the problems with existing studies is that many different strengths and types of ginkgo preparations have been used, and it is unclear if there is an optimal and safe dosing regime. However, Germany recently approved ginkgo extracts (240 mg a day) to treat Alzheimer's disease and this may give some guide. Too often it is incorrectly presumed that all herbal remedies are safe, and it should be noted that ginkgo can cause stomach bleeding, especially when taken with aspirin.[14]

Physical exercise can increase cerebral blood flow, which may in turn be beneficial for mental function. There are certainly studies that demonstrate that exercise can improve memory and mood, though none have specifically shown that exercise prevents dementia. There are many valid reasons for embracing physical exercise; it would not be surprising if it turns out that dementia prevention is another benefit.

NUTRITION

Vitamin B_{12}, Vitamin B_6 and folate—the role of homocysteine

Vitamin B_{12} (cobalamin), vitamin B_6 (pyridoxine) and folate play vital roles in effective DNA synthesis and normal brain metabolism. These B-group vitamins act as catalysts in chemical reactions in which homocysteine is converted to methionine, and dietary deficiencies can result in a build-up of serum homocysteine. High levels of homocysteine have been linked with Alzheimer's disease, vascular dementia, cerebrovascular disease and cognitive impairment in general. In addition, vitamin B_{12}, vitamin B$_6$ and folate deficiencies are known to cause depression and other neurological syndromes. What is unclear at present is whether these associations reflect a causal mechanism between high levels of homocysteine and dementia. There is some evidence that high levels may exacerbate cognitive impairment after acute stroke, so there may be an additive effect. Certainly, homocysteine provides another link between Alzheimer's disease and cerebrovascular disease, but the extent to which it may be responsible for either condition is not known.[15]

Probably the most important issue is that there is a simple treatment for preventing high levels of homocysteine. A diet rich in green leafy vegetables, low-fat dairy products, citrus fruits and juices, wholewheat bread and dry beans can significantly lower levels of homocysteine. Since 1998, the US Food and Drug Administration (FDA) has required the addition of folic acid to enrich breads, cereals, flours, corn meals, pastas, rice and other grain products, but it is too soon to know whether this will reduce the rate of dementia. In Australia, where folate enhancement of grain products does not routinely occur, folate supplements could be considered. In individuals with normal folate levels but elevated homocysteine levels, low dose folate supplementation (50 micrograms daily) should suffice, while individuals with folate deficiency may require up to 5 milligrams daily until the deficiency is overcome before reverting to a lower dose. Of course, vitamin B$_{12}$ replacement is required if that vitamin is deficient.

Unfortunately there have been no randomised controlled studies of folate supplementation for the prevention of dementia. While it is speculative to suggest it as a reasonable prevention strategy, it is unlikely to be of harm and may have other cardiovascular benefits. Folate supplementation could be regarded as a universal preventive measure suitable for the entire population.

Fish

A recent French study has reported that the consumption of fish at least once a week reduces the risk of dementia by one-third over a seven-year period. This protective effect may be explained by the omega-3 polyunsaturated fatty acids contained in fish oils, which have a protective effect against cardiovascular disease and hence on the vascular risk factors implied in vascular dementia and Alzheimer's disease. They could also have a specific effect on brain development and neuroprotection, though this is unproven. Another factor may be education; this was found to exert an independent effect, with more highly educated older people eating more fish.[16]

Caffeine

Whether or not this is the best place to deal with caffeine is debatable—while for some of us caffeine is a major nutrient, there may be argument about it! There has long been evidence in the test tube that caffeine may have a potential role in treating Alzheimer's disease. Caffeine belongs to a family of chemicals that includes drugs such as propentofylline, currently in the final pre-licensing stages by the USFDA as a treatment for Alzheimer's disease. Propentofylline acts by modulating the activity of glial cells in the brain. Caffeine itself has been shown to stimulate nerve cells to take in more choline, the building block for acetylcholine, the most important neurotransmitter for memory function. Caffeine also blocks receptors for adenosine, another neurotransmitter, a function thought to be of potential therapeutic benefit in Alzheimer's disease.

In July 2002, the first clinical evidence that caffeine consumption might be associated with lower rates of Alzheimer's disease was published in a case control study. The study has numerous weaknesses but does point to the need for larger, prospective studies. At this stage, however, there is insufficient evidence to recommend the use of caffeine to prevent Alzheimer's disease.[17] It should be remembered that caffeine can have adverse effects on sleep and on the heart, and can increase anxiety.

SUMMARY

Traditional strategies to prevent disease have focused upon disease elimination. In the case of dementia, a delay in the onset of the disease may have a preventive effect as potential victims may die of other disorders before they develop dementia. An understanding of risk and protective factors for dementia is required before any preventive strategies can be undertaken. Universal prevention strategies are those that can be applied to the whole population.

Table 2.1 summarises the various universal dementia prevention strategies and comments on the strength of evidence and potential tolerability. Most universal strategies are easy to apply, have a wide range of health benefits and few, if any, drawbacks. Examples include dietary changes to improve antioxidants in our food, continuing physical exercise and continuing education. The extent to which these strategies may reduce the risk of dementia is unclear, but they are unlikely to harm.

Table 2.1 Summary of universal dementia prevention strategies

Risk factor	Prevention strategy	Strength of evidence 0 = no evidence 1 = weak 2 = modest 3 = strong 4 = proven	Tolerability 0 = intolerable 1 = low 2 = moderate 3 = very tolerable
Age (oxidative metabolism)	Antioxidants—vitamin C and E rich foods (not supplements)	2: Needs placebo-controlled prospective trials, could delay dementia onset	3: Unlikely to harm and likely to have other health benefits
High serum homocysteine	Folate rich foods, possibly supplements	2: Needs placebo-controlled prospective trials; approximately doubles risk of Alzheimer's disease	3: Unlikely to harm and likely to have other health benefits
??Low cerebral blood flow	Ginkgo biloba	1: Possibly reduced risk of Alzheimer's disease though mechanism unclear	2: Usually well tolerated but may cause bleeding
Low brain reserve, cognitive inflexibility	Life-long education, physical exercise, mental activity	2: In later life needs placebo-controlled prospective trials to establish effect; in early life more longitudinal cohort studies	3: Unlikely to harm and likely to have other health benefits

CHAPTER 3

PREVENTION OF DEMENTIA II

IN CHAPTER 2, PREVENTION STRATEGIES that are applicable to everybody were considered. In this chapter, strategies that are applicable either to individuals at increased risk of dementia or to individuals already experiencing mild symptoms of possible dementia (mild cognitive impairment) are considered.

SELECTIVE DEMENTIA PREVENTION STRATEGIES

Selective prevention strategies are directed towards individuals at high risk with established risk factors for a disease. Common examples include weight reduction in overweight people to reduce the risk of coronary artery disease and diabetes, smoking cessation to reduce the risk of lung, heart and blood vessel disease, and increased calcium intake in people with osteoporosis to reduce the risk of fractures. Some dementia prevention strategies in this category may be useful for everybody, not just those with risk factors for dementia, and I indicate those which are most promising. Not all established dementia risk factors currently have effective preventive strategies.

GENETIC FACTORS

Genetic factors are known to be causative in most early onset (presenile) dementias, and there is now mounting evidence that they contribute in a major way to the development of late onset Alzheimer's disease. Genetic factors and age are the two main established risk factors for Alzheimer's disease. Unfortunately, there are currently no recognised preventive strategies that can directly reduce the genetic risk.

Familial Alzheimer's disease

Most of the highly publicised advances in the genetics of Alzheimer's disease have come from the study of very rare families with so-called Familial Alzheimer's disease (FAD). FAD is an autosomal dominant disease, which means that 50 per cent of each generation develop Alzheimer's disease, usually between the ages of 40 and 60 years. Causative mutations on chromosome 14 (presenilin-1 gene), chromosome 1 (presenilin-2 gene) and chromosome 21 (amyloid precursor protein gene) have been found in these families. Hints that chromosome 21 could be implicated came with the finding that there was a higher rate of Down syndrome, a genetic disorder due to abnormalities on chromosome 21, in the family history of Alzheimer patients, and with the observation that the majority of persons with Down syndrome who survive to late adulthood develop dementia.

In individuals with early onset Alzheimer's disease, diagnostic DNA testing will confirm whether it is a familial form, although in 30 per cent of cases no mutation will be found. Predictive testing of family members can then be undertaken, if desired, to determine which individuals have the mutation and thus allow for genetic counselling. Currently, there are no specific treatments available for these family members, and in the absence of such treatment, the take-up for predictive testing is low.[1] (The potential for gene modifying therapies is discussed in Chapter 13.)

Late onset Alzheimer's disease

The vast majority of cases of Alzheimer's disease are due not to a mutation in a single gene, but rather reflect the presence of a number of genetic risk factors (polymorphism) that interact with environmental factors. Inheritance through this type of genetics does not follow simple rules that allow for neat predictions of chance. When relatives of patients diagnosed with Alzheimer's disease ask what their chances are of getting Alzheimer's disease, the question is not easily answered. The longer we live the more likely we are to develop dementia; by the age of 100 most people are likely to be dementing. If we consider only the first-degree relatives of patients who develop Alzheimer's disease by the age of 85 years, there is a threefold to fourfold increased risk of their developing Alzheimer's disease, as compared to the general community. This translates to a lifetime risk somewhere between 16 and 20 per cent, which may be quite worrying. In considering this risk, however, it is necessary to take into account the likelihood of a person surviving to a certain age. Using actuarial tables in combination with these risk percentages, it has been calculated, for example, that a first-degree relative surviving to the age of 78 years has a less than 10 per cent chance of having developed Alzheimer's disease. Overall, less than one-third of the risk is realised in the normal lifespan. Putting it in these terms will reassure many relatives, particularly those who are concerned that they may develop Alzheimer's disease at a younger age, which can be shown by similar calculations to be an extremely rare event. For second-degree relatives such as grandchildren, the risk of developing Alzheimer's disease is probably less than twice the overall population risk, though there has been only limited research on this to date.

Only one gene, that for apolipoprotein E (apoE), has been definitely associated with late onset Alzheimer's disease. Apolipoprotein E, a protein synthesised in the liver and brain, is involved in lipid metabolism and tissue repair. There are three common forms of apoE, known as apoE2, apoE3 and apoE4, the genes for which are on chromosome 19. In 1993, it was observed that the frequency of apoE4 in patients with Alzheimer's disease was greater than that found in age-matched controls. This has been confirmed in numerous studies around the world. Further, the risk is higher in people who are homozygous for apoE4 (that is, have two apoE4 genes—one inherited from each parent) than in those who are heterozygous (only one apoE4 gene). These findings suggest that apoE4 status increases the risk of developing Alzheimer's disease, but the mechanism is as yet unknown.

Current opinion is that the apoE4 genotype determines when rather than whether a person develops Alzheimer's disease. Carriers of apoE4 appear to develop Alzheimer's disease earlier, with estimates suggesting that at most some 50 per cent of people who are homozygous for apoE4 will develop Alzheimer's disease within their lifetime. There is also some suggestion that carriers of the apoE2 gene may have some protection from getting Alzheimer's disease, a suggestion supported by the high rates found in centenarians.

Consensus statements from Alzheimer's Disease International and Alzheimer's Association/National Institute of Aging in the United States have concluded that there is no current role for apoE genotyping in the prediction of risk of developing Alzheimer's disease or in the diagnosis of Alzheimer's disease. In diagnosing Alzheimer's disease, while the presence of the apoE4 gene may increase diagnostic accuracy in persons with dementia, its absence has little value in endorsing or refuting the diagnosis. Thus the benefit of testing seems negligible. Of course, it is possible that in the future a better understanding of how the apoE4 protein influences the pathophysiology of Alzheimer's disease may result in potential preventive strategies that target apolipoprotein E.[2]

VASCULAR RISK FACTORS

It has long been recognised that factors that increase the risk of stroke, the so-called vascular risk factors, also increase the risk of vascular dementia. What has been surprising in recent years is the discovery that these factors also increase the risk of Alzheimer's disease.[3] Common susceptibility genes may be one of the reasons for this. Many vascular risk factors can be modified by simple lifestyle changes, but despite this there has been little research that has directly examined their preventive potential.

Hypertension

High blood pressure is probably the single most important risk factor for stroke and vascular dementia. This is certainly the case in midlife where a history of high blood pressure in combination with heart disease or diabetes increases the risk of vascular dementia up to sixfold, and also Alzheimer's disease by two- to threefold.[4] Two important studies have indicated that benefits still accrue when treatment for high blood pressure is commenced in old age. The Syst-Eur trial found that older people with high blood pressure who were treated with antihypertensive medication for two years had a reduced incidence of stroke and dementia compared with those randomly assigned to placebo. The incidence of dementia was reduced by 50 per cent, but intriguingly most of the cases were of Alzheimer's disease rather than vascular dementia, as might have been expected.

Extrapolating from this study, over five years, the treatment of 1000 hypertensive people would prevent nineteen cases of dementia.[5]

The PROGRESS study involved 6105 individuals in Asia, Australasia and Europe with a history of stroke or transient ischaemic attack (mini-stroke); they were treated with anti-hypertensive therapy alone, or in combination with diuretic medication, or placebo, and followed up for four years. While there was a 12 per cent reduction in cases of dementia this was largely related to vascular cases, which was in keeping with the overall reduction in stroke, by up to 43 per cent depending on the regimen used.[6]

These findings indicate that optimal treatment of high blood pressure is an important preventive measure for dementia, though the degree of specificity for any particular type of dementia remains uncertain. Whether similar benefits can be obtained by other lifestyle measures that are known to reduce high blood pressure—reducing salt in the diet, weight control, increasing physical fitness and optimising alcohol intake—is yet to be seen. Commonsense would suggest that these should form the cornerstone of a lifestyle intended to reduce the risk of dementia.

Smoking

Smoking is strongly associated with cardiovascular disease, peripheral vascular disease, stroke and vascular dementia. For some years, studies appeared to suggest that smoking had a mild protective effect against Alzheimer's disease, possibly from the nicotine, but recent larger, better quality studies have shown that smoking is associated with up to double the risk of Alzheimer's disease. The relationship may not be as simple as it appears at first glance however, because smoking appears to interact with other risk factors, including alcohol, gender and genetic factors, to both increase and decrease the chances of getting Alzheimer's disease. More research is needed to tease out what may be happening.[7]

At this stage, however, encouraging older people to stop smoking should be considered as part of a strategy to reduce the incidence of cognitive impairment. Another consumer warning that could be placed on cigarette packets might be 'Remember to stop smoking to remember'. There are many reasons to stop smoking—and dementia risk is yet another.

Diabetes mellitus

Diabetes mellitus is associated with moderate cognitive deficits and brain changes that may be referred to as diabetic encephalopathy. Recent studies have shown that type 2 diabetes, which usually develops in later life and is believed to be strongly influenced by diet and obesity, increases the risk of Alzheimer's disease by around one-and-a-half to twofold, and of vascular dementia by over twofold. In individuals with the apoE4 gene, type 2 diabetes increases the risk by five-and-a-half-fold. Both vascular and non-vascular factors are likely to play a role in dementia in diabetes, where mixed aetiology is likely.[8]

Atherosclerosis and reduced cerebral blood flow

It is probably self-evident that a reduction in blood flow to the brain will adversely affect brain function. It is well known that blockage of the main arteries to the brain can result in strokes and hence vascular dementia. More subtle reductions in cerebral blood flow that occur in people with cardiovascular and other circulatory problems might also be damaging. Atherosclerosis (hardening of the arteries) damages the carotid and vertebro-basilar arteries, the main blood vessels supplying the brain. This results in a build-up of platelets, blocking the arteries and acting as a source for small blood clots (emboli) to pepper the brain. Atrial fibrillation, in which there is an irregular heart rate, can have the same effect. Both conditions frequently result in transient ischaemic attacks (TIAs). For many years, low dose aspirin has been prescribed for its ability to stop platelets from sticking together, which has been shown to reduce the risk of stroke and TIAs. There is also evidence that aspirin can slow the progression of vascular dementia; however, no studies have examined whether it may actually prevent dementia. As aspirin is a potent cause of stomach irritation and bleeding, unless other vascular risk factors demand its use to reduce the risk of stroke, it cannot be recommended as a routine preventive measure for dementia until strong studies demonstrate its effectiveness.

Coronary artery bypass surgery

Between 50 and 80 per cent of patients undergoing coronary artery bypass surgery become confused after the surgery and have cognitive impairment at discharge from hospital. While many have questioned the importance of this cognitive deterioration, there is now mounting evidence that impairments are still found in 42 per cent of patients five years after surgery. Because persistent cognitive impairments are associated with early post-operative confusion, efforts to reduce post-operative confusion may prevent such impairments. However, it is unclear whether the effect predisposes to dementia, and further research is required to determine if this is the case.[9]

NUTRITION

Cholesterol

There are a number of links between cholesterol and Alzheimer's disease. Major studies have shown that people with cholesterol levels above 6.5 in midlife increase their risk of Alzheimer's disease in later life at least two-and-a-half-fold. In addition there is a convergence of research, for apolipoprotein E, which is associated with an individual's risk of developing Alzheimer's disease, carries cholesterol in the brain. It also promotes the formation of the amyloid plaques that are a hallmark of Alzheimer pathology.[10] There is also some laboratory research suggesting that high levels of cholesterol cause the body to produce more amyloid precursor protein and hence more beta-amyloid.[11]

Statins are a class of drugs that lower levels of low density lipoprotein (LDL) cholesterol—the type most strongly linked with coronary artery disease and stroke—by blocking a liver enzyme essential for cholesterol production. Examples include fluvastatin (Lescol, Vastin), simvastatin (Lipex, Zocor), atorvastatin (Lipitor) and pravastatin (Pravachol). While statins reduce the risk of stroke by 29 per cent, several studies have shown that they also reduce the risk of dementia.[12] Researchers at Boston University presented the most promising of these studies at the American Academy of Neurology's annual meeting in April

2002. This study examined the effects of statins on 2581 people—912 people with probable or definite Alzheimer's disease and 1669 of their family members who did not have the disease—from more than 800 families over six years. It showed that the use of statins cut the risk of developing Alzheimer's disease by as much as 79 per cent, even in people who were genetically predisposed to the disease. This effect was found to be greatest in African Americans.[13] While these findings are very promising, prospective randomised controlled studies are required to confirm whether statins have a preventive role.

There is mounting evidence that cholesterol metabolism plays a role in the development of Alzheimer's disease, although its relative importance in the overall picture remains unclear. With the current controversy surrounding the subsidisation of statins for the treatment of high cholesterol on the Australian Pharmaceutical Benefits Scheme, it is unlikely that dementia prevention will be added to the list of indications until there is much stronger prospective randomised placebo-controlled research to support their use. Another aspect that requires further attention is whether cholesterol levels currently regarded as normal are in fact potentially harmful. In other words, are there potential benefits in lowering everyone's cholesterol level, not just for those whose levels are high?

High calorie and high fat diets

A recent report has indicated that individuals who eat a high calorie (more than 1870 kilocalories per day) and high fat diet have more than double the risk of Alzheimer's disease—but only if they are carriers of the apoE4 gene. Non-carriers were not at increased risk with such a diet. This is a good example of the importance of the interaction between genetic and lifestyle risk factors.[14] Another recent study from Sweden, published in July 2003, has found that women who are overweight in later life have an increased risk of Alzheimer's disease. For every 1.0 increase in Body Mass Index at age 70 years, the risk of Alzheimer's disease increased by 36.1. This effect was not found in men.[15] Given the other recent dietary findings, these results are not surprising.

GENDER: THE ROLE OF HORMONE REPLACEMENT THERAPY

While there does not appear to be an overall difference in the rates of dementia between men and women, there are differences in the types of dementia. Some studies show that women have slightly higher rates of Alzheimer's disease and that men have higher rates of vascular dementia.

The higher rate of Alzheimer's disease in women may relate to a combination of increased longevity, increased survival with the disease, and some increase in intrinsic vulnerability. The latter may link with evidence that oestrogen protects the brain from damage, possibly by regulating nerve growth. It has been observed in some studies that women who are taking oestrogen as hormone replacement therapy (HRT) after the menopause have approximately a 30 per cent lower risk of developing Alzheimer's disease, particularly if they have been taking it for at least ten years. As these studies were not designed specifically to determine whether HRT might prevent dementia, a number of other risk factors for dementia related to lifestyle and education were not controlled for, and it could be that these other factors explain the difference.[16]

There are large trials underway in the United States designed to address this issue. One of these studies, the Women's Health Initiative Study, involving 16 600 women taking a combination of oestrogen and progesterone, which was due to be completed in 2005, was abruptly halted in July 2002 as a 26 per cent increase in breast cancer, and higher rates of heart disease, stroke and blood clots, were recorded after 5.2 years of treatment. Even the risk of dementia was increased. The researchers found that the risks were outweighing the benefits. Within days an expert committee from the Australian Therapeutic Goods Administration recommended that combined hormonal replacement therapy not be used in long-term replacement.[17]

These findings may not affect other studies in progress that involve the use of oestrogen alone. The Women's International Study of Long Duration Oestrogen after Menopause—Cognition (WISDOM-COG), to be completed in 2006, will provide information about the effects of HRT on cognitive ageing. The Preventing Postmenopausal Memory Loss and Alzheimer's with Replacement Estrogens Study (PREPARE) and the dementia component of WISDOM-COG (to be completed in 2003 and 2009 respectively) will address the question of whether oestrogens can delay or prevent dementia. These ongoing clinical trials will also be the first to study the effects of oestrogen in women with natural versus surgical menopause, on cognitive ageing and risk of dementia.

Several trials of oestrogen in the treatment of women with Alzheimer's disease have been negative, but this may simply mean that the oestrogen was given too late. In fact, a recent study demonstrated that the protective effect of oestrogen was greater in former than in current users, suggesting that oestrogen loses its effects in the pre-clinical stages of Alzheimer's disease. Another possibility recently suggested by research from Oxford University is that folate supplementation may need to be given with the oestrogen replacement for it to be effective.

The pros and cons of oestrogen-only HRT are still heavily debated, even without consideration of the potential to prevent Alzheimer's disease. The other benefits of oestrogen-only HRT include an overall 44 per cent reduction in mortality over five years, and up to 50 per cent reduction in hip fracture, against the previously mentioned concerns of increased risk of breast cancer and deep vein thrombosis. For post-menopausal women, any decision to use HRT will need to consider carefully these potential risks and benefits; at this stage there is insufficient evidence to support its routine use for the prevention of Alzheimer's disease alone.[18]

The increased risk of vascular dementia in men has mainly been attributed to lifestyle factors rather than to any inherent male factor, although evidence that androgens may increase the risk of cardiac disease suggests there may be indirect male factor effects. Some recent research has found that older men with higher levels of free testosterone had better memory and cognitive function. This may suggest that testosterone could play a protective role against cognitive decline, but this idea is speculative.[19] Lifestyle factors will be discussed later.

INFLAMMATION: THE ROLE OF ANTI-INFLAMMATORY MEDICATION

Both Alzheimer's disease and vascular dementia are characterised by inflammatory responses that are believed to contribute to the death of nerve cells. Epidemiological studies have identified a reduced risk of Alzheimer's disease in people with arthritis and leprosy being treated with anti-inflammatory drugs. Longitudinal studies have shown that the consumption of anti-inflammatory medications for two or more years reduces the risk of Alzheimer's disease by up to 80 per cent, but has no effect on the risk of vascular dementia.[20]

In contrast, treatment studies of Alzheimer patients with low dose steroids (prednisone) and non-steroidal anti-inflammatory medication (celecoxib and indomethacin) have failed to demonstrate a significant effect. It is possible that the dose of prednisone was too low to be beneficial; there are also concerns that, to be effective, anti-inflammatory medication may need to be given very early in the course of the disease, possibly before the individual is symptomatic. Of interest is the fact that one of the more commonly prescribed anti-inflammatory drugs, ibuprofen, has been shown to have an effect on amyloid metabolism. To date, however, there have been no controlled trials of ibuprofen on the prevention or treatment of Alzheimer's disease. Currently underway in the United States is a large study called the Alzheimer's Disease Anti-inflammatory Prevention Trial (ADAPT) that will run over seven years to better address this question.[21]

As anti-inflammatory medications have many side-effects, including stomach irritation, bleeding and anaemia, they cannot be recommended for either prevention or treatment of Alzheimer's disease until sound placebo-controlled studies have been published.

OCCUPATIONAL EXPOSURES: ELECTROMAGNETIC RADIATION, FUMIGANTS/DEFOLIANTS

The search for occupational risk factors for dementia has yielded few results. The large French PAQUID study did not find any occupational risk factors for Alzheimer's disease.[22] While another study found that occupations involving the use of electric motors close to the body have around three times greater risk of developing Alzheimer's disease, two other studies found no relationship. The occupations included electrician, machinist, carpenter, sheet-metal worker, toolmaker, seamstress, typist and welder. If that study's findings were to be confirmed, better shielding of electric motors might have a protective effect.[23]

One Canadian study has found that occupational exposure to fumigants/defoliants increased the risk of Alzheimer's disease by over fourfold. This is biologically plausible, as the chemicals involved have an adverse effect on neuronal activity. Again, if this finding were to be supported by other studies, better protective clothing in the handling of these chemicals would be beneficial.[24]

DELIRIUM (ACUTE CONFUSIONAL STATE)

Older hospitalised people are at high risk of developing delirium, otherwise known as an acute confusional state. In most cases there are identifiable medical causes—infections, reduced brain blood supply, side-effects of medication, dehydration and recent surgery, to name a few. While delirium is a sign of severe illness and is associated with increased mortality, treatment of the underlying causes usually results in recovery of mental function. Dementia is a risk factor for delirium and it is well established that when persons with dementia become ill, their confusion increases. Many caregivers anecdotally report that after such an episode their loved ones fail to regain their previous level of function.

There is now mounting evidence that non-demented persons who become delirious have an increased risk of developing dementia. Some do not fully recover, others recover only to decline in the following few years. Although the most likely explanation is that incipient dementia was present at the time of hospitalisation and the delirium represented a breach of symptom threshold, there is also a possibility that delirium may cause permanent brain damage. It is thus unclear whether strategies to prevent delirium could be regarded as selective strategies for high-risk individuals, or as indicated strategies for individuals with early symptoms.

Sharon Inouye from Yale University has demonstrated in a series of elegant studies that the rate of delirium can be reduced in the hospitalised elderly by a combination of strategies that include early identification of high risk individuals, rehydration, reality orientation, mobilisation and mental stimulation. Results of the long-term effects of these strategies on the development of dementia are not yet available. If it can be demonstrated that dementia risk is reduced, it will add further weight to the implementation of delirium prevention programs in hospitals.[25]

INDICATED DEMENTIA PREVENTION STRATEGIES

Indicated prevention strategies target individuals who are showing early symptoms of disease but may not reach full criteria for the disease, or are not yet showing any damage from the disease. Common examples include coronary artery bypass surgery to treat mild angina so that heart attacks are prevented, excision of pre-malignant skin lesions and removal of pre-cancerous bowel polyps. Currently there are no proven strategies that prevent the progression of early symptoms of mild cognitive impairment to dementia.

COGNITIVE IMPAIRMENT

Many terms have been used to describe states of mild cognitive disturbance that are not severe enough to qualify for the diagnosis of dementia. These include 'mild cognitive impairment', 'age-associated memory impairment' and 'benign senescent forgetfulness'. Each is defined in slightly different ways and each is associated with an increased risk of developing dementia. Mild cognitive impairment (MCI) has received most attention recently and is described in more detail in Chapter 4.

Persons with MCI will progress to Alzheimer's disease at a rate of 10 to 15 per cent per year, compared with healthy control subjects who convert at a rate of 1 to 2 per cent per year. A research group at the Mayo Clinic in the United States, observing a group of subjects with MCI for more than ten years, has demonstrated a conversion to Alzheimer's disease of up to 80 per cent. Survival rates for MCI subjects over a seven-year period are midway between those of normal elderly people and Alzheimer patients. Although therapies are being developed that might prevent progression of MCI to Alzheimer's disease, there is no evidence at present to support prescribing therapeutic agents. However, intensive research is now being undertaken in several multicentre treatment trials involving more than 4000 subjects.[26]

This research highlights one of the key ethical issues in this area. Defining MCI as a pathological state has opened the door to the pharmaceutical industry to develop agents to treat it and thus becoming a driving force behind attempts to maintain MCI as a diagnostic entity. Critics of the current application of the MCI concept believe there is still insufficient evidence to warrant its distinction from the other age-related cognitive changes previously described. It is not that it is doubted that such states exist, only that their current identification is too imprecise. Using current criteria, the use of drugs in the MCI population to improve memory and prevent Alzheimer's disease is likely to result in the treatment of a significant number of normal elderly.

Another issue highlighted by this dilemma is the prospect that while a successful treatment for a person with MCI may be defined as non-progression to Alzheimer's disease, it may not result in any meaningful improvement in the individual's memory and hence may result in that person spending more time living with a significant disability.

Depression in old age

Prospective studies of whether depression may be aetiologically linked to cognitive decline and dementia have yielded variable results. Statistical analysis of pooled data has found that depression was associated with an increased risk of subsequent dementia. Older people with depression have a twofold to threefold risk of developing dementia—but it is quite possible that their depression is part of their evolving dementia, which may not become apparent for a few years. Depression in early to middle adulthood has been found to be associated with an increased risk of vascular dementia, but not of Alzheimer's disease, 25 years later. This finding may have been mediated by vascular risk factors.[27] There is no evidence that effective treatment of depression alters the risk of dementia.

Some unproven factors

Over the years many and various environmental factors have been suggested as potential 'causes' of dementia, and of Alzheimer's disease in particular, but research has failed to substantiate the claims. Here I mention some of the prominent ones.

Aluminium

Since the 1960s there have been repeated claims that aluminium may be important in the development of dementia. Aluminium is known to be toxic to the nervous system. Chronic renal dialysis patients developed 'dialysis dementia' due to the high levels of aluminium that accumulated during the dialysis process. Further, there was some evidence of increased levels of aluminium in the brains of persons with Alzheimer's disease, and some animal studies found that high levels of aluminium may provoke Alzheimer-type changes in the brain. These claims led to many people throwing out their aluminium cooking utensils. However, numerous epidemiological studies have failed to demonstrate any consistent association between levels of aluminium in diet, water or medication (antacids) and Alzheimer's disease. In addition, the pathological changes found in the brains of dialysis dementia patients are quite different to those of Alzheimer's disease. Aluminium seems an unlikely major factor at this point.[28]

Viral infections

Viruses are implicated in so many diseases that it is not surprising they have been considered as potential factors in Alzheimer's disease. The discovery of the HIV virus, and its ability to cause dementia many years later, added impetus to the search. Other viruses, such as the herpes zoster virus that causes shingles, are sequestered in nerve cells for decades after initial exposure before becoming symptomatic. This means that viral exposure in child-hood, or possibly in utero, could theoretically be involved. So far research has been largely negative, though one study did find higher rates of herpes simplex infection in Alzheimer patients. Much stronger evidence is required before any concerns about viral infections should be expressed.[29]

Food-borne toxins

Several rare neurological conditions have been linked with the intake of food-borne toxins found in legumes in Africa, India and Guam. In Canada, an outbreak of a neurological disorder similar to Alzheimer's disease occurred amongst people who had eaten mussels contaminated with demoic acid. These examples provide evidence that food-borne toxins could potentially be implicated in Alzheimer's disease, but no specific toxins have been identified that affect the broader population.[30]

Bacterial infection

Researchers from Washington University, St Louis in the United States have discovered that common bacteria responsible for urinary infections, wound infections and food poisoning (*Escherichia coli* and *Salmonella*) can sometimes produce amyloid protein which increases their resistance to antibiotics. This raises the question as to whether bacteria may play a role in amyloid production in the brain. One study has reported evidence of pneumonia-causing *Chlamydia* bacteria in the brains of persons who have died with Alzheimer's disease, but this is a long way from establishing any link with the development of the disease. Much more research is required.[31]

SUMMARY

Although there are now numerous factors identified with increased risk of dementia, it is fair to say that the two factors with the strongest impact are currently the hardest to change—age and genes. This conclusion is emphasised by research that has shown that persons with superior health over the age of 85 years are not protected from developing Alzheimer's disease. In the case of Alzheimer's disease, altering most of the other factors may delay the onset of dementia rather than eliminate it, while attention to vascular risk factors offers better hope of elimination of vascular dementia. Delay of onset may be as good as cure, however, providing other terminal diseases in old age such as heart disease and cancer continue unabated—but, there is no guarantee!

In Table 3.1 I summarise the various selective and indicated prevention strategies, and comment on the strength of evidence and potential tolerability. Some strategies are easy to apply and have a wide range of health benefits and few, if any, drawbacks. Other strategies, for example anti-inflammatory medications and hormone replacement therapy, may have potentially greater effect but are currently unproven and have significant adverse effects. In between are strategies that are indicated in specific circumstances, for example high blood pressure and cholesterol, where the treatments may have adverse effects and their potential to prevent dementia is not entirely proven. As new studies are published every few months in this field, you should consult your doctor for specific advice.

Table 3.1 Summary of selective and indicated dementia prevention strategies

Risk factor	Prevention strategy	Strength of evidence 0 = no evidence 1 = weak 2 = modest 3 = strong 4 = proven	Tolerability 0 = intolerable 1 = low 2 = moderate 3 = very tolerable
1. Selective strategies—people at high risk			
Gender: oestrogen deficiency in women	Hormone replacement therapy in post-menopausal women	2: Needs placebo-controlled prospective trials; only 30% risk reduction	2: Other health benefits are currently a stronger indication and there are adverse effects
Inflammation: early effects of Alzheimer's disease	Anti-inflammatory medication in individuals at high genetic risk of Alzheimer's disease	2: Needs placebo-controlled prospective trials; about 67% risk reduction suggested	1: High rates of adverse effects—anaemia, gastric irritation and bleeding
Hypertension	Antihypertensive medication and diet in people with high blood pressure, history of stroke or TIA	4: Vascular dementia, but only modest reduction 2: Alzheimer's disease	2: Most agents have the potential for adverse effects but there are other health benefits
Smoking	Stop smoking	3: Vascular dementia 2: Alzheimer's disease	3: Unlikely to harm and likely to have other health benefits

Cholesterol	Statins, diet in those with high cholesterol; ?? benefits universal	2: Needs placebo-controlled prospective trials for Alzheimer's disease and vascular dementia	2: Most agents have the potential for adverse effects but there are other health benefits
Atherosclerosis	Antiplatelet medication (aspirin)	1: Vascular dementia 0: Alzheimer's disease	1: High rates of adverse effects—anaemia, gastric irritation and bleeding
Diabetes mellitus	Diet, weight loss, better control of diabetes	1: Both vascular and Alzheimer dementia—in both cases risk is increased but strategy may not work	3: Unlikely to harm and likely to have other health benefits
Head injuries	Approved helmets for those at risk—boxers, bike riders	2: Potential to reduce dementia is modest	2: Some find helmets too restrictive
Delirium	Multifaceted delirium prevention programs for hospitalised older people	0: Trials underway; unproven cause of dementia	3: Unlikely to harm and likely to have other health benefits
Electromagnetic radiation	Better shielding of electric motors in workplaces	1: More studies required	2: Unlikely to harm but may have economic effects
Fumigants/defoliants	Better protective clothing for workers at risk	1: More studies required	2: Unlikely to harm but may have economic effects

2. Indicated prevention—individuals with early symptoms or signs of dementia

Mild cognitive impairment	Cognitive-enhancing drugs	3: Strong evidence of risk but no evidence of benefit from strategy; trials underway worldwide	2: Most agents have the potential for adverse effects in 20-30%

The great appeal of substances such as *Ginkgo biloba* and vitamins is that they are not prescription drugs. They are also relatively cheap and easily available. However, little is known about the side-effects of supplements taken in large doses over a prolonged period, and there is some evidence that supplements do not work in the same way as naturally occurring vitamins in food. The consumer should be cautious in their use.

We are on the cusp of dementia prevention strategies that may have some meaningful outcomes; future prospects are discussed in Chapter 13.

CHAPTER 4

THE SYMPTOMS AND COURSE OF DEMENTIA

IN MOST CIRCUMSTANCES, DEMENTIA is a progressive condition that results in an evolving pattern of symptoms, behaviours, functional impairments and disabilities. The nature of an individual's presenting symptoms and the pattern of their evolution will provide clues to the underlying type of dementia. For example, Alzheimer's disease tends to develop almost imperceptibly and progress gradually over a course that may run, on average, for six to twelve years. Vascular dementia has a more varied presentation and course, but a common variant is of relatively sudden onset followed by a stepwise decline over a somewhat shorter timespan than seen in Alzheimer dementia. Because for most persons dementia is a chronic disorder, it is useful to view its course in stages according to the severity of the disease process. Note that these stages should be viewed as only a rough guide, since they are mainly based on the course of Alzheimer's disease, not the other types of dementia. Further, some people may have some features from one stage and other features from an earlier or later stage.[1] There are also many different symptoms of dementia, as listed in Table 4.1.

PRE-DEMENTIA: MILD COGNITIVE IMPAIRMENT

As with most illnesses, dementia has no set pattern of early symptoms. Presentations can be quite varied, and often are recognised only retrospectively. Furthermore, early symptoms may be subtle and attributable to many causes, a problem accentuated by dementia's relatively slow progression. Currently we have limited knowledge of these earliest symptoms of dementia, and of how

Table 4.1 Symptoms of dementia

Memory impairment
Disorientation and confusion
Impaired language skills
Behavioural changes
Psychological symptoms—depression, anxiety and psychosis
Impaired judgement, insight and decision making
Intellectual decline
Impaired functional capacity
Impaired social function

they might be distinguished from normal ageing and other mental conditions. As pre-dementia merges almost imperceptibly with early dementia, the symptoms are discussed in more detail in the next section.

EARLY OR MILD DEMENTIA

People with early dementia are able to function independently in most aspects of their life. Long-acquired social skills can compensate for their impairments, so it is not surprising to find that many acquaintances are unaware of there being any problem at all. In fact, a mistake that some family members make after a dementia diagnosis has been made is to 'cottonwool' the dementing person and not allow them to lead as normal a life as possible.

Short-term memory impairment is usually the most prominent early symptom of Alzheimer-type dementia. Such impairment results in the afflicted person having difficulty in remembering recent events—where they put the keys an hour ago, what their daughter told them on the phone last night, what they did last weekend. Contrary to popular belief, most people are aware of deterioration in memory. The majority, however, lack insight about the extent of their deficits and tend to deny that it is really impacting on their lives. When interviewed with family members present, upraised family eyebrows often accompany denial of the severity of the problem. More remote memories from childhood, adolescence and early adulthood are relatively unaffected in the early stage of dementia, yet in most cases probing questions will reveal mild deficits, for example, minor mistakes in the chronology of their life history. Some people are very insightful about their memory loss and are acutely aware that it is abnormal. In my observation, the increased community awareness of dementia and Alzheimer's disease has resulted in more people presenting for assessment with a subjective awareness of their memory deficits.

> For several years, Mary's family had noticed she was becoming more forgetful. She frequently lost her keys and on two occasions had had to have her front door locks changed. She seemed to forget telephone conversations that she had with her daughter, Alice. In one instance this resulted in Alice waiting for her mother at the shopping centre for over an hour, to have Mary say later that she must have been mistaken, as she hadn't been told about the arrangement. Despite these occurrences, Mary seemed to be coping quite well by herself, albeit more slowly and with fewer social outings. Alice wasn't too concerned—after all, her mother was 81 and 'Don't we all lose our memory as we get older?' It was only when Mary started to accuse her daughter of stealing her belongings when she visited her that Alice wondered whether there was something more seriously wrong. It was at this point that Alice decided to approach her mother's GP about her concerns.

This is a typical case history in which there has been a presumption that persistent memory impairment is due to age-related changes. It is only when other behavioural changes are superimposed upon the memory disturbance that action is taken. Hopefully, improved community awareness about dementia will result in more people being referred for assessment as soon as memory changes are detected. Short-term memory can be affected by numerous conditions, some of which include depression, stress, deafness, infections, medications, tumours, cerebrovascular disease and inflammatory disorders, in addition to age-related changes to memory function. Distinguishing normal ageing from the effects of such conditions, and from dementia, is the main aim of dementia assessment.

Word-finding difficulties (aphasias) are also common, particularly with types of dementia that mainly involve the parietal and temporal cortical areas of the brain, for example, Alzheimer's disease and frontotemporal dementia. Aphasia results in difficulties in finding the correct word for an object or the name of a familiar person. It can be manifested in several ways—the person might say 'the thing that holds the watch on the wrist' instead of 'watchband', or will simply stop mid-sentence and express frustration with their efforts to find the right word. Others will report that they can no longer reliably remember the names of friends and acquaintances. There is also some recent evidence that for some years before Alzheimer's disease becomes apparent, the dementing person may have difficulties in understanding speech when there is a lot of background noise or other competing signals. For people who have English as a second language, aphasia may show itself in other ways.

Angelo migrated to Australia from southern Italy in the 1950s to work on the Snowy Mountains Hydroelectric Scheme. He spoke no English when he arrived, but after a couple of years learned enough to get by, and by the 1960s spoke fluently, albeit with a thick Italian accent. At the age of 73, Angelo's short-term memory began to decline. To the consternation of his family, he also started to have trouble finding the correct English word when he spoke, substituting an Italian word instead. Within a few years, Angelo was speaking a hybrid of English and Italian and seemed to understand conversations in Italian best. This created problems for his grandchildren, who did not speak Italian.

There is a general rule with dementia—'last in, first out'. Languages and other skills acquired later in life are usually the first skills lost as the dementia progresses. Thus people from a non-English speaking background characteristically lose their English language skills before their native tongue is affected.

Personality and behavioural changes are initially very subtle and usually put down by family members and friends to age, stress, depression and sundry other causes. Dementias that involve the frontal lobe of the brain—frontotemporal dementia, vascular dementia and sometimes Alzheimer's disease—are particularly prone to this presentation. The slightly reserved, considerate person may start telling risqué jokes and committing repeated *faux pas*. The responsible, conservative investor may gradually take increased risks on the stockmarket. The placid, agreeable husband may become irritable, argumentative and tempera-mental. An outgoing, sociable wife may lose interest in going out with her friends and become generally apathetic in her outlook. The meticulously groomed woman may start going out with poorly applied cosmetics and stained clothing.

In other cases, rather than a change to the opposite there is an exacerbation of pre-morbid personality traits. The temperamental, verbally abusive husband turns to physical violence. The quiet, shy person becomes withdrawn and subdued. The easily worried, emotional person becomes persistently anxious, clingy and inse-cure. The suspicious, guarded loner becomes overtly paranoid.

Such personality and behavioural changes will clearly have an impact upon the person's lifestyle, resulting in family tensions and disruption of long-standing friendships. Sometimes the family doctor is consulted, though often nothing specific can be found. It is usually only when other symptoms occur and the diagnosis of dementia is made that the family becomes aware that the changed personality and behaviour is part of the dementia. At times irreparable damage may be done to relationships before the cause becomes clear. This is one situation where an early assessment by a psychiatrist or neurologist to clarify the cause of the changes may possibly limit the damage to family and social relationships.

Depression may be an early feature of dementia. Sometimes the clinical depression shows no hint of dementia and responds to antidepressant therapy, the other symptoms of dementia emerg-ing months or years later. At other times, repeated efforts to treat what appear to be depressive symptoms are unsuccessful or are only partially effective. In these situations, apathy due to frontal lobe impairment may often obscure the dementia diagnosis. In a third situation there is a mix of depressive symptoms and memory changes, and it may be unclear for some time whether the memory problems are due to the depression or to early dementia. The circumstance where depression is mistaken for dementia (pseudodementia) will be discussed later.

At 68 Mark seemed to have reached a dead end. He had retired from the public service when he was 63 and, together with his wife Annette, had initially led a very active lifestyle with overseas travel, voluntary work and plenty of exercise. He was a passionate golfer, playing with his wife and friends several times a week. Over the previous two years, he had gradually given up all these pursuits, preferring instead to sit around at home all day. No matter how hard Annette and his friends tried to encourage him, he remained disinterested. He just couldn't understand their concerns. He seemed happy but had lost all motivation. There were no marital problems, though Annette was starting to lose her patience with him. His doctor had prescribed several courses of antidepressant medication with no effect. At this stage, he was referred for assessment by a psychogeriatrician.

It is not surprising that this type of history would suggest depression as a possible cause of Mark's symptoms. Indeed, I would be concerned if he hadn't been treated with reasonable trials of antidepressant therapy. In the early stages, damage to the frontal lobes of the brain can be very difficult to distinguish from depression and investigations may be inconclusive. This is often very frustrating for family carers, who do not know where they stand.

Acute confusional episodes include symptoms of disorientation, perplexity, agitation, visual hallucinations and delusions (irrational false beliefs). Typically they are transient, usually lasting minutes to hours, though sometimes for a few days. In early dementia, these episodes tend to occur mainly in vascular dementia, dementia with Lewy bodies and dementia associated with Parkinson's disease.

Such episodes are possibly most commonly associated with the transient confusion and hallucinations that may occur when waking from a dream at night. This is an extension of the normal phenomenon of 'hypnogogic hallucination' that many of us have experienced on awakening—a state in which it may take seconds to minutes to realise that we are still dreaming. The difference is that the acute confusional episode usually lasts longer, and the person experiencing it may take some time to be reassured, as they tend to have poor insight into what has happened. Also, such episodes tend to start happening repeatedly.

Another common scenario is that in which a person becomes temporarily lost and disoriented when in a familiar locale, for example when driving or shopping. Sometimes this may overlap with short-term memory lapses, such as when a car is left in a shopping mall carpark and cannot be found. Again, with assistance from another person or after a short period of reflection, the confusion often settles.

Post-operative confusion after routine surgery may also be the first sign of early dementia. Frequently there is an underlying medical reason for the confusion (for example, infection, blood loss), but the mere fact that confusion has occurred at all is often a warning sign. Usually the confusion settles within days with appropriate treatment, but sometimes it becomes clear to the family that full recovery hasn't occurred. In many cases, the confusion has merely added to subtle signs of memory or personality change which had been noticed before the surgery. Occasionally there are no pre-operative symptoms, and the possibility that there has been an adverse intra-operative event must be considered.

> At 85, Daisy had become rather frail. Her bones were weakened by osteoporosis and arthritis and her mobility was poor. She also had high blood pressure, diabetes and asthma, and suffered from constipation, which led to her being prescribed ten different medications each day by a variety of medical specialists and her GP. Despite these problems, her family felt she was 'reasonably alert' and only occasionally forgetful. It came as no surprise, however, when she fell and fractured her hip. Twenty-fours after surgery, her son was called by the hospital to be informed that Daisy was severely confused, agitated and calling out. Her state improved over the next fortnight but she remained more forgetful, less alert and indecisive. Her family was convinced that something must have happened during the operation.

Another occasional situation where acute confusional states may herald the appearance of dementia is illustrated by the following case.

> David and Joan were travelling through Europe on a coach tour. One night at 3 am an agitated Joan rudely awoke David. She told him that something strange had happened to their home—the bathroom had been moved. David had enormous difficulty convincing her that they were in a hotel room in Europe. She seemed to really believe that she was home in Sydney but eventually settled with reassurance. David didn't think much more about it as the next day Joan was back to her normal self and when he told her what had happened she could barely recall it, so they both just shrugged it off as a bad dream. A few nights later, in a different hotel, Joan again

woke David in the middle of the night with the same concern. This time she wasn't easily reassured, and also expressed the belief that possibly the neighbours were responsible and were trying to trick her. After an hour, David became so concerned that he called for the hotel doctor, who arranged for a hospital assessment. Joan's confusion settled within hours and no significant acute medical problems were detected. Joan was advised to have a more detailed examination when she returned to Australia.

As more retirees travel, this type of situation is occurring more frequently. Of course, disorientation and confusion in unfamiliar surroundings are common problems that can spoil holidays for both dementing people and their carers. Taking precautions when travelling, such as always having a familiar carer present, keeping the travel time as short as possible, taking familiar bedside objects to put into the new bedroom, having plenty of rest periods, maintaining hydration and exercise and avoiding alcohol, can all help to minimise difficulties.

MODERATE OR MIDDLE STAGE DEMENTIA

Probably the major feature that distinguishes moderate dementia from mild dementia is the clear need for the dementing person to be provided with some level of assistance to allow them to maintain their function in the community as near as possible to the level they enjoyed before the onset of the dementia.

Memory and orientation

By the moderate stage of dementia, memory function is severely affected. Memories of recent events are very poorly retained, though in some people verbal and visual reminders or cues may elicit some recall. Mentioning a friend's name might be a reminder of a visit to their home. Showing a picture of a relative might remind them of a birthday. If the event that has just occurred has great emotional significance, recall is likely to be better. For example, the death of a spouse in the previous week is likely to be remembered to some degree, while a routine bus trip would not be. This was demonstrated graphically in Japan a few years ago after a major earthquake. Many dementing nursing home residents could remember the earthquake, but not recent, mundane, day-to-day events.

Remote memories are also more overtly affected. While the dementing person will still dwell in the past, their reminiscences are repetitive and lacking in detail. The chronological sequence of past events is now certainly disrupted. Their marriage may occur before they were born, the birthdays of children are entangled and ages are a guesstimate. Even knowledge of where their marriage occurred, their place of employment and details of important world events such as World War II are usually impaired.

Disorientation in time is a constant. There is little chance of knowing the day, date or month of the year reliably, though they may know the year. The usual response is along the lines that 'all days seem the same' or 'it really doesn't matter what day it is'. Orientation in place will depend on where they are. Usually disoriented in unfamiliar surroundings, in their own home they will as a rule know where they are. Trips to new or only vaguely familiar places may provoke anxiety and confusion. However, repeat visits to a new place that is perceived as being friendly and relaxing, such as a dementia day care centre, will usually quell anxiety, and the dementing person may attain a degree of orientation to it. There are exceptions to this, as noted in the following vignette.

Raymond had been diagnosed with Alzheimer's disease for four years and was cared for by Jennifer, his wife. She had been able to look after him without too much concern until one day he demanded to be taken home—when he was sitting in his own lounge room. Taken aback, Jennifer initially didn't know what to say but after reassuring him and showing him around the house, he settled down. Wisely, Jennifer had Raymond checked by their local doctor, who could find no evidence of any acute medical problem and advised her that it was likely to be part of the dementing process. These episodes started to happen on a regular basis and it became apparent that Raymond believed that he still lived in the house they used to occupy in a different suburb in the early years of their marriage. On one occasion he became so insistent that Jennifer took him to the site of their long-demolished first home to convince him he was mistaken. Eventually she discovered that the only way to mollify Raymond was to take him out in the car, drive him around the block and pretend that they had arrived home.

This type of strategy doesn't work for everyone but is well worth trying. It is a good example of 'going with the flow' rather than trying to convince the dementing person that they are mistaken.

Acute confusional episodes where there may be marked disorientation associated with behavioural changes, hallucinations and paranoia developing over hours to days are now likely to occur when there is an infection or other acute medical condition.

Language and calculation

Naming difficulties are more noticeable in everyday speech. Names of familiar people and common objects are regularly stumbled over. Less obvious to the casual listener but quite apparent to family and friends is the growing impoverishment of speech. The content has less detail, fewer spontaneous comments are made and much of what is said is repetitive. Indeed, repetitive utterances can cause enormous distress to carers, particularly when they take the form of a question. Despite the carer giving an answer, the same question may be asked minutes later . . . and again and again and again. This is called 'speech perseveration'. Another example is the same response being given repeatedly to different questions. Multilingual persons often use several languages simultaneously and are largely unaware they are doing so. The most recently acquired languages continue to erode the quickest.

Comprehension is also more severely affected. What carers may interpret as poor memory may in fact be poor comprehension of what has been said. Complex commands may be misunderstood, sometimes to the extent that a hearing deficit is suspected and a hearing aid considered. In similar vein, comprehension of written material is also poor. This, in combination with diminished concentration, memory and motivation, usually results in a marked reduction of time spent in reading. Carers will note that the same page in the book has been 'read' for days or weeks.

Simple calculations may no longer be reliably completed, particularly without pen and paper. This is most noticeable in shopping, where the dementing person often relies completely on the honesty of the shop assistant to give the correct change. Even given their date of birth and the current date, it is also unlikely that they will be able to calculate their age.

Executive and intellectual function

Executive function, largely a function of the frontal lobes of the brain, can be equated with managerial skills. A decline in intellectual skills is noted by an inability to solve day-to-day problems, learn new skills (for example, how to operate a new appliance) or appreciate abstract aspects of relationships. Organisational and planning abilities become progressively impaired. The dementing person may repeatedly say they are going to do something but never get around to doing it. In this way, hobbies and other life-long interests are progressively abandoned. Skills acquired earliest are usually retained longer—'first in, last out'. Judgement and insight about their own capacity may be poor, with a failure to recognise their own limitations. This may also extend to judgements about others, as seen in the following case.

> Julie had always been friendly and enjoyed company. Despite her dementia, she still lived alone with support from family and neighbours. When a young man with a hard luck story knocked on the door and offered to do some odd jobs, she felt obliged to help out. She paid him $30 to do $10 worth of shopping. Unsurprisingly, he returned regularly, usually after pension day, and was paid well each time for very small jobs. She felt unable to refuse, despite having a nagging feeling that she should. A pensioner, she had always been careful with her finances. Her family started to become concerned when Julie kept asking to borrow money. They noted that several large sums of money had been withdrawn from her bank accounts shortly after pension day. Julie told them a vague story of a destitute young man who had been helping her.

I regularly assess dementing people in their homes and am constantly amazed at how trusting most people are with strangers. While this makes my job easier, it is also apparent how vulnerable many dementing people are to fraudulent tricksters.

Self-care and functional capacity

It is during this stage that capacity for self-care declines; it is particularly noticeable in people who live alone. Personal hygiene, dressing, cooking, shopping, financial management and social skills become impaired. Usually the dementing person doesn't recognise the need for assistance, due to their impaired judgement and insight, and may only grudgingly accept help. Many persons with moderate dementia are living alone in the community with minimal or no assistance. Almost inevitably this is achieved by accepting a reduction in their standard of living, for example, by living in dirty conditions, by wearing soiled clothing, by eating little food of dubious freshness, by socialising minimally or by having financial problems through forgetting to pay bills.

Mavis had lived alone since her husband died ten years earlier. She had always looked after herself without needing to call on her daughter Jane, who lived interstate, though she maintained regular phone contact and visited each year. For some years Mavis had been getting more forgetful. She and Jane put it down to age now that she had reached 78. During her previous visit, Jane had noticed that the usually impeccable home was rather untidy (as was Mavis herself), that the customarily well-stocked refrigerator contained plenty of milk (much of it out of date) and only a few other odds and ends, and that several unopened power and water bills lay on the kitchen table. Mavis had explained this by saying she had been 'sick with a virus' and was just about to do it all. After Jane had helped her mother clean the house, pay the bills and restock the fridge, she suggested that maybe it was time that she accepted some regular help with the shopping and housework. It was like a red rag to a bull. Mavis angrily told her daughter that she didn't need any help and that if this was 'the sort of way that you are going to treat me' she would be better off not visiting. She quickly calmed down, however, and by the time Jane returned home all was forgiven. Over the next six months Jane phoned at least weekly and often every few days as she became increasingly concerned about the extent of her mother's forgetfulness and poor self-care. She quickly gained the impression that unless she reminded Mavis to shop and pay bills, little would be done. An earlier than usual visit was arranged, not that Mavis noticed. Jane was shocked to see how messy her mother's home had become and by her apparent lack of concern. Mavis was wearing a heavily soiled dress and smelled as if she hadn't bathed for weeks. Despite Jane's phone calls, the fridge was again bare and unopened bills lay on the table. As before, Mavis claimed she had just recently had a 'virus', but otherwise she felt okay and didn't need any help.

This is a common type of scenario, leading family members to difficult choices about when and how to insist that some type of community service be introduced to help the dementing person cope at home. It frequently results in referrals to an Aged Care Assessment Team, which ensures that the dementing person is thoroughly assessed, an accurate diagnosis is obtained and the prognosis is outlined.

For some carers it comes as a surprise to be told that the changes in self-care and function are due to dementia, not age. Knowing what the future is likely to hold, however, both the dementing person and the carer are in a better position to plan, even at this relatively late stage of the disease.

When the person with dementia is living with a carer, usually a spouse, many self-care and functional capacity issues are effectively concealed from the outside world as the carer gradually takes on more and more tasks. Sometimes the transfer of responsibilities is achieved almost imperceptibly over some years, and without any dramas. For example, the dementing person may be gently reminded to have a shower; clean clothes will appear after the shower and the dirty ones be removed surreptitiously and dressing will be monitored to ensure the clothes are put on correctly. Often the degree of dependence only comes to light in a crisis, for example, when the carer becomes acutely unwell, and it comes as a great surprise to friends and other family members that the dementing person is so incapacitated.

Of course, the dementing person's transition from independence to partial dependence doesn't always go smoothly and can become the source of much conflict with the carer. Issues that often lead to disputes include financial management, driving, personal hygiene and social activities. These are discussed in more detail in later chapters.

Behavioural changes

It is in this stage of dementia that behavioural changes become more marked, occurring to a significant degree in approximately 50 per cent of cases. Studies have demonstrated that challenging behaviours and associated psychological symptoms are strongly associated with carer stress and placement of the dementing person in residential care. Not all changes of behaviour are a problem. Often an explanation that the behaviour change is part of the dementia allows the carer to tolerate it. At other times the behaviour itself is not abnormal, it is just occurring in the wrong place or at the wrong time. Other behaviours can be more of a challenge.[2]

Activity disturbances

Wandering occurs in 30 to 40 per cent of cases, and may become a serious concern. 'Wandering' is an all-encompassing term covering a broad range of behaviours that involve a change in the physical activity of the dementing person and/or the ability to find their way back home. In moderate dementia, wandering behaviours mainly involve an element of disorientation—the dementing person becomes lost and attempts unsuccessfully to find their way home. Sometimes they use commonsense and get a cab or ask for help; more frequently a good Samaritan notices their confusion and provides assistance. Often this occurs after a considerable period of walking. At other times the desire to walk simply increases without necessarily involving any disorientation. Long daily walks around the neighbourhood occur, often to the concern of family members, who fear the dementing person will either get lost or accidentally walk in front of a car. Sometimes the walking is aimless and associated with general restlessness; at other times there is a particular purpose. One type of purposeful wandering can occur in the situation described in the earlier vignette, where Raymond might start wandering from his current home in a search for his previous home.

Underactivity can also occur and is usually associated with general apathy and amotivation. Some dementing people take to their bed for no apparent reason and appear happy to have carers provide for their every need. This can be very frustrating for the carer.

Aggressive behaviour

A particular complication of hallucinations and paranoid delusions is the increased risk of aggressive behaviour. This may range from verbal abuse and irritability to actual violence. Occasionally serious assaults may ensue. Treatment of the psychosis reduces the risk of dangerousness. Aggressive behaviour also can occur without psychotic symptoms through a coarsening of the pre-morbid personality, low frustration tolerance, depression or disinhibition. Often aggression only occurs when assistance is required with personal care. The dementing person may simply be uncooperative; sometimes actual physical aggression occurs. Aggressive behaviour is one of the more difficult behaviours for carers to cope with, but many bear with it for a considerable time before requesting help.

Tamara had always regarded her husband Rupert as a gentleman. Throughout their marriage he had been courteous, caring and supportive to her and their children. As his Alzheimer-type dementia unfolded, some early signs of per-sonality change became quite pronounced. Four years after being diagnosed, Rupert was now easily irritated and would swear at Tamara when frustrated, using four-letter words she had never heard from him before. Sometimes he would push her, which on several occasions resulted in bruises. This marked change in Rupert's personality and behaviour was extremely distressing for Tamara, but she felt that to tell her chil-dren, friends or doctor about what was happening would be a betrayal of her husband. So she kept it to herself, largely by severely limiting her social contacts and giving a range of increasingly improbable excuses for her bruises to her children and friends. Eventually, after a particularly distressing incident, she realised that she needed help and consulted her doctor.

This is not an unusual story. Wives in particular often tolerate quite disturbed behaviour for a long time before seeking help. Embarrassment, obligation and sometimes fear prevent many from getting assistance. Of course, other carers do not tolerate even relatively minor behavioural changes and seek help at an early stage.

Sleep disturbance

One of the effects of neuropathological changes in the brainstem is a disruption of the sleep–wake cycle. Sleep patterns progres-sively deteriorate as the dementia worsens, more so in people who have previously been poor sleepers. Sleep periods become shorter, shallower and more frequent, so it becomes common to have naps during the day and periods of wakefulness at night. At its extreme, day–night reversal of sleep patterns can occur. Carers often face a similar situation to mothers of restless babies, becoming sleep deprived themselves with consequent irritability, poor concentration and symptoms of depression.

Disinhibited behaviour

Disinhibited behaviours occur where there has been an impairment of the psychological processes that restrain the expression of instinctual drives. In dementing people this usually occurs due to frontal lobe damage. There are certain behaviours that we learn very early are socially inappropriate—picking our noses in public, walking down the main street without clothes, touching another person without consent, telling complete strangers intimate personal details, and so on. When these behaviours occur in dementia, family and friends are often very distressed. Disinhibited sexual behaviours can be particularly upsetting. Most persons with moderate dementia do not engage in regular sexual activity, but occasionally libido appears to increase and their partner may be repeatedly propositioned every day. Occasionally sexual molestation of carers may occur, particularly in residential care. Often this takes the form of fondling breasts and bottoms. In some cases the behaviour may represent an inappropriate way of trying to express intimacy needs.

Psychological symptoms

Often linked with behavioural changes, it is useful to conceptualise psychological symptoms separately because they are often quite distressing to the dementing person whereas behavioural changes usually only bother other people. It is not surprising that moderate dementia should cause a wide range of psychological symptoms, for it is during this stage that the impact of declining cognition and function really becomes noticeable to the dementing person. There is evidence that psychological symptoms are associated with neuropathological and neurotransmitter changes in various parts of the brain, though there is a lack of consensus about specific changes. Even though their impaired insight may serve to limit the impact, most dementing people will, if given the opportunity, express their difficulties in understanding their changing world in a variety of ways.

Misinterpretations, illusions and psychosis

Misinterpretations and illusions become prevalent and take many forms. Relatives are accused of stealing misplaced objects, familiar people are misidentified, normal neighbourhood noise is misconstrued as machinery, and friends are accused of talking about them behind their back. This especially occurs at night when sensory stimuli are less, and in unfamiliar surroundings. Another important factor may be the presence of a visual agnosia due to the dementia, which results in the person being unable to recognise common objects despite otherwise normal eyesight. Sometimes a simple demonstration of where lost objects are located, or an explanation of the misinterpreted event, allied with reassurance, will result in the dementing person's acceptance of being mistaken—although the problem is likely to recur.

At other times no amount of explanation or reassurance will alter their beliefs. There is usually a sense of persecution and suspiciousness. In these circumstances, the beliefs have become delusional and the dementing person is regarded as having a psychosis. One particularly distressing type of delusion is illustrated in the next case.

Joseph and Eva had been married for 53 years in a devoted relationship in which neither had contemplated life without the other. They met in a refugee camp after World War II, having both narrowly escaped death in the Holocaust. After marrying, they resettled in Australia and decided that they were not prepared to have children. Throughout their marriage they kept to themselves and had few friends. At the age of 82, Joseph had a mild stroke in which he became briefly confused and unsteady on his feet. Subsequently, Eva noticed that he started to have memory lapses, which worsened six months later after another mild stroke. Of greater concern, he became irritable and intermittently started to accuse Eva of having an affair with a neighbour. Her reassurances only served to anger him. She felt devastated by the turn of events. Fortunately her GP was very supportive and managed to convince Joseph to take an antipsychotic drug; after a few weeks his delusions lessened and he stopped persecuting Eva.

This type of delusion is known as 'morbid jealousy'. Unfortunately there is a high risk of physical assaults in these situations, so control of the delusions with medication is crucial. Morbid jealousy can occur in many situations apart from dementia and is not always due to a psychosis. Some people are just inherently jealous and while they may not actually believe their partner is unfaithful, they constantly query their fidelity and may even search for signs that an affair has occurred.

Visual and auditory hallucinations may also occur, but usually in association with delusions. People and animals may be seen, neighbours' conversations may be overheard from quite a distance, strange machinery noises perceived. It is sometimes difficult to know whether there is any factual basis to the experience. For example, it is not uncommon for the person who believes he can overhear his neighbours to be living in an apartment with thin walls through which noises are easily transmitted. Another issue is that hallucinations are much more likely to occur in people with hearing and visual deficits. Sometimes the 'noises' are really tinnitus, but this explanation is not often readily accepted; usually the dementing person prefers a delusional interpretation, such as the neighbours using a new electronic gadget to keep him or her awake at night.

Depression

Depressive symptoms are common during this stage of dementia, occurring in up to 50 per cent of middle stage dementias. A far lower percentage experience actual clinical depression. Depression may occur as a psychological reaction to declining mental function, as an exaggeration of pre-morbid traits, or as an inherent part of the dementia due to changes in brain neurotransmitters. Depression may be difficult to diagnose in a dementing person but should be suspected if they wish to die or have suicidal ideas, where there has been an otherwise unexplained sudden decline in function or change in behaviour (for example, aggression or reduced appetite), or the person is tearful for no apparent reason. As mentioned previously when discussing early dementia, distinguishing depression from frontal lobe apathy is also not easy.

Anxiety

Symptoms of anxiety are also common and often occur in association with depression. Anxiety symptoms are more likely to occur in a pre-morbidly anxious person. Intense fear of abandonment by the carer is an especially challenging situation in which the dementing person won't let their carer leave them for even a few minutes without becoming very agitated. This can lead to the carer feeling trapped. When the anxious person with dementia lives alone, frequent phone calls to family and friends for reassurance are likely to occur. This may happen many times every day, to the intense frustration of the recipients. The anxiety often improves dramatically in company, so an element of loneliness is likely. This presents the obvious solution of living with others, either family, friends or in a hostel, but there is generally a surprising degree of resistance to the suggestion.

Social function

In moderate dementia, independent social functioning has all but disappeared. While there may be a facade of normality, this is usually achieved by the efforts of an attentive carer or sensitive friends. Alone, the dementing person is liable to make errors while shopping, travelling and banking, and they usually require the goodwill of service providers to get through. For many people, attempts to function independently in social situations are so anxiety provoking that social activities are largely abandoned. For others, the loss of initiative and organisational skills largely prevent participation in social activities without someone else to arrange it. Friends who do not understand why they are no longer contacted by the dementing person may incorrectly feel they are being snubbed and respond by ceasing to make contact themselves. This lack of social interaction may increase boredom and depression. It is often noted that when an organised social activity is regularly arranged the dementing person perks up.

SEVERE OR LATE STAGE DEMENTIA

By this stage of dementia, there is no semblance of independent function and the majority of persons with severe dementia are in residential care. Maintenance at home usually requires 24-hour care from family, friends and community support services. The level of care required is so intense over such a long time (usually a year or two) that, in the absence of an intercurrent illness, almost all persons with severe dementia eventually spend some time in a nursing home.

Memory and orientation

There is now very severe to profound memory impairment. There is virtually no recall of recent events and past memories are fragmentary and imprecise. Concentration is extremely poor and the person is very distractible on many tasks. In addition to being disoriented in time, there is now disorientation in place and, as the dementia worsens, disorientation to self, with the person being unable to cite their name. In married women this often announces itself initially when they start to respond with their maiden name.

Confusional episodes associated with any medical illness, medications, environmental changes, pain, constipation and sundry other causes are the rule rather than the exception in severe dementia.

Language

Language skills are rapidly lost. Speech becomes increasingly impoverished, with the use of simple sentences or phrases, and very concrete interpretations of questions. There is little evidence of spontaneous conversation, with the majority of spontaneous utterances being requests for some form of help. Often the same words or phrases are repeated over and over again (perseveration). Many sufferers eventually completely lose their speech (become aphasic). Speech is replaced by various noises, somewhat like the range of sounds that pre-verbal infants use. In a similar fashion to infants, many of the sounds have meaning that perceptive carers are able to understand. And, like the noises made by pre-verbal infants, the loud repetitive utterances of late stage dementia can be extremely stressful for carers.

Anne had severe Alzheimer's disease and had been in the nursing home for a year. For the past six months her speech had been limited to a few words. Yet she would chatter continuously for hours at a time in a loud high-pitched voice. Most of the time she would repeat the same sounds over and over again—'Da-da-da-da-da', screeches, or sometimes discernible words. Her noisiness was very disruptive to other residents and staff. Visitors complained, as did neighbours. It got to the stage that staff avoided her as they found her 'chattering' so stressful.

Comprehension appears to be more slowly eroded, though it is necessary to communicate using simple language slowly and often with associated gestures.

Executive and intellectual function

In severe dementia there is very limited intellectual function. There is no semblance of capacity to organise and plan, the dementing person being completely dependent on others. Decision making is restricted to very simple choices and often impeded by poor judgement. Insight is minimal. There is often no recognition of the extent of incapacity and the person may become very angry and distressed about being unable to do things when they want to. This is one of the factors contributing to some of the challenging behaviours in this stage of dementia that are discussed later. Yet a partial ability to learn simple things may remain for a surprising amount of time, a capacity that allows carers to modulate some behaviour. Also, musical appreciation may be retained to the extent that the types of music that the person enjoyed in the past may still evoke enjoyment.

Self-care and functional capacity

During this stage of dementia, the dementing person progresses from requiring assistance to toilet, bathe, eat and dress to being fully dependent on a carer to do these things for them. Self-care skills are rapidly lost without regular practice, thus it is not unusual to see a marked decline in function after a prolonged illness such as pneumonia. Due to this tendency, carers are always encouraged to allow the dementing person to do as much for themselves as possible, though the dilemma may be that this takes an inordinate amount of time. Urinary and later faecal incontinence is universal, though this progresses in stages from occasional nocturnal incontinence, to incontinence that responds to regular toileting by staff, to complete incontinence requiring 24-hour continence pads. Swallowing problems are common, particularly in persons with vascular dementia, and may result in recurrent bouts of pneumonia caused by inhalation of food and stomach acid. Others simply stop eating, which raises the vexed question of tube feeding, discussed in Chapter 12. If the dementing person doesn't die of an intercurrent illness (most frequently pneumonia, stroke or heart attack), eventually the ability to walk is lost and they become initially chairbound and then bedbound.

Behavioural changes

Challenging behaviours reach a peak around the period of transition from moderate to severe dementia. Each of the behaviours described for moderate dementia continues to occur in severe dementia, though as functional impairment becomes more marked, and physical function declines, they tend to diminish. It should also be remembered that these behaviours are not universal, although as dementia progresses non-verbal means of communication increase. Some behaviours in severe dementia are mainly a form of communication but the challenge to carers (and part of the reason for the term 'challenging behaviour' rather than 'problem behaviour') is to determine the meaning.

Activity disturbances

While overactivity prompts most concern in severe dementia, activity levels generally reduce and many people become quite inert without prompting from carers. This underactivity can be a major problem, contributing to sleep disruption and boredom. General restlessness and aimless wandering are the predominant overactivity disturbances. One situation that causes a lot of concern is where a person who is unable to walk safely without assistance insists on walking alone and repeatedly falls over. Physical restraints can be applied to stop the falls, but this has the consequence of increasing their agitation and distress. Some people who are bedbound will writhe around so forcefully that they throw themselves out of bed.

Uncooperative behaviours

Many challenging behaviours in severe dementia reflect a clash between an insightless dementing person who wants to do or not do something and a carer who is trying either to prevent the dementing person from endangering themselves or to assist them with a function. As the dementing person's functional capacity diminishes, there are more and more occasions where hands-on physical assistance is required. Some people quite enjoy the help and are cooperative, others object to the loss of autonomy, or feel embarrassed, or maybe simply don't like the particular person helping them or the way they are being helped. Sometimes even well-meaning staff can inadvertently be rough. Uncooperative behaviours can range from stubborn resistance to verbal and physical aggression. The following case is typical.

Ricardo had severe vascular dementia and a hemiparesis from a recent stroke. He was completely dependent on the nursing home staff for all his basic care. He was completely incontinent of urine and faeces but whenever the nursing staff tried to change him he became very agitated, pushing them away and sometimes striking them. It reached a stage where the staff were reluctant to change him even though they knew this was untenable. Eventually they found that he was more cooperative with male staff, and with those who spoke his native Spanish.

Finding the right approach for the individual can be a challenge for both professional and informal carers. Sometimes the most unexpected things work. It is important that carers do not give up in their efforts to try different strategies, though each new strategy should be given a reasonable trial before being abandoned as unsuccessful.

Eating behaviour

Eating behaviour changes in a variety of ways in moderate to severe dementia but 'refusal to eat' causes greatest concern, especially when it is associated with weight loss, which tends to happen in most persons with severe dementia anyway. 'Refusal to eat' encompasses a range of issues and in many cases is an inaccurate description of what is happening. The coordination required to use knives and forks to eat declines due to the dementing process, and sometimes food left untouched simply reflects this loss of function. Most persons with severe dementia need to be fed, but some spit out the food, push it away or won't open their mouths. As dementia becomes more severe, the ability to eat falls off. The masticatory process becomes uncoordinated, chewing may be ineffective, tongue movements may fail to prepare the food bolus to be swallowed, and the swallowing reflex may be incompetent. These are all good reasons for apparent food refusal. Other factors that may contribute to 'refusal to eat' include the quality of the food, ill-fitting or absent dentures, inability to see the food due to poor eyesight and the lack of a social milieu that encourages eating. Many carers become concerned that food refusal may be due to the dementing person 'giving up' in a depressed mood, and this may occasionally be the case. I investigated 'refusal to eat' with Henry Brodaty and colleagues in a nursing home study in Sydney, and found that depression was not commonly associated with it.[3]

Other changes in eating behaviour, which may become apparent in earlier stages of dementia, include predilections for certain food such as sweets and chocolates, overeating, eating of inedible objects (pica) and an alteration in taste which may be related to a reduced sense of smell.

Disinhibited behaviour

In severe dementia, the types of disinhibited behaviour that cause concern are varied. Intrusiveness and rummaging through other people's possessions are common. Usually the dementing person has no idea that they are in someone else's room. Confrontations may occur, with violent outcomes. Vocally disruptive behaviour with repeated calling out for assistance or attention is a particularly distressing behaviour for staff and residents. Inappropriate sexual behaviours that tend to occur later in the dementia include exposure and masturbation in public.

Psychological symptoms

It is difficult to tell what the psychological processes of a person with severe dementia who is unable to speak coherently or write might be. At least for these reasons, studies of the symptoms of anxiety, depression and psychosis show a decline in prevalence as dementia progresses. Interpretation of non-verbal communications suggests that psychological reactions are still occurring but what they are is difficult to ascertain. Smiles, cries, frowns, winces all convey meaning and almost certainly reflect underlying emotional states.

Social function

While independent social function is no longer possible, social interactions remain important. In a non-threatening environment that caters for the limitations in their function, most persons with severe dementia thrive. Supervised dance, exercise, music, games and involvement with simple chores often provide surprising insights into quiescent abilities. Some people, of course, have never enjoyed social activities and won't change. Others are too distractible to stay for long.

ADVANCED DEMENTIA

Many dementing people die before they reach the stage of advanced dementia, particularly if they have other significant health problems. By this stage the dementing person is completely dependent on carers for all aspects of daily living and has almost certainly been in nursing home care for some years. Language skills are lost and many are mute. Memory function is virtually impossible to test. Most are unable to stand or walk without assistance, many are unable to sit up properly. Due to their lack of activity, passive exercises are essential to prevent contractures of arms and legs, and routine pressure care is required to prevent the development of bed sores. Most nursing homes have good pressure care routines but if residents with advanced dementia are transferred to hospital for any reason, there is a high risk that they will return with bed sores. (Acute hospitals seem to have difficulty in implementing pressure care effectively alongside all the other demands made on their staff.) Feeding difficulties are almost universal and many people with advanced dementia are unable to swallow safely. This again raises the issue of tube feeding, discussed in Chapter 12. Urinary and faecal incontinence is the rule.

Most dementing people die from infections (pneumonia, influenza), cardiac arrest or stroke.

SUMMARY

Most types of dementia are gradually progressive as they course through mild, moderate, severe and advanced stages. This means that the symptoms of early dementia differ from those found at later stages. Apart from impairments in memory and orientation, the other symptom domains of dementia include language and calculation, executive and intellectual function, behaviour, psychological reactions, self-care and functional capacity, and social function.

CHAPTER 5

TYPES OF DEMENTIA

THERE ARE OVER 100 established types of dementia, but most of them are extremely rare. In this chapter I will describe the four main types of dementia seen in clinical practice—Alzheimer's disease, vascular dementia, frontotemporal dementia and dementia with Lewy bodies, which account for 90 to 95 per cent of all cases—and a number of the less common types, as listed in Table 5.1.

In the previous chapters I have outlined the common risk factors for dementia and described the clinical features, albeit with a particular focus on Alzheimer's disease. Here my focus is on what is understood about why these disorders occur, and the specific features that distinguish them from each other.

Apart from vascular dementia, most of the dementias are categorised as neurodegenerative disorders because, essentially, they involve the progressive degeneration and death of nerve cells. There is now mounting evidence for a common theme uniting these disorders. In a nutshell, neurodegenerative disorders are fundamentally caused by the abnormal accumulation of insoluble proteins in the brain. These proteins are toxic and exert a deleterious effect on selective nerve cells, impairing their function and eventually leading to cell death. The abnormal proteins also affect synapses (spaces) between nerve cells, hence the chemical information between cells might not be transmitted properly and nerve circuits might be interrupted.[1] This is a fast moving area with new discoveries happening almost every week. I concentrate on what seems to be reasonably well accepted by the scientific community rather than on what remains speculative.

Table 5.1 Types of dementia

Common dementias (90–95%)

    Alzheimer's disease

    Vascular dementia

    Dementia with Lewy bodies (DLB)

    Frontotemporal dementia

Uncommon dementias (5–10%)

Other neurodegenerative diseases

    Parkinson's disease

    Progressive supranuclear palsy

    Cortico-basal degeneration

    Creutzfeldt-Jakob disease (CJD)

    Huntington's disease

    Familial British dementia (FBD)

Traumatic causes

    Head injuries

    Subdural haematoma

Tumours

    Brain tumours—primary and secondary

Infections

    HIV/AIDS dementia complex

    Neurosyphilis

    Chronic meningitis

    Viral encephalitis

Toxic, metabolic and endocrine causes

    Thyroid disorders

    Vitamin B_{12} and folate deficiency

    Metabolic disorders—chronic kidney and liver failure

    Chronic drug intoxication, e.g. long-term anti-epileptic medication

    Alcoholic dementia

Other

    Normal pressure hydrocephalus

    Auto-immune disorders, e.g. temporal arteritis

    Anoxic brain damage, e.g. after cardiac arrest

Figure 5.1 The neuron

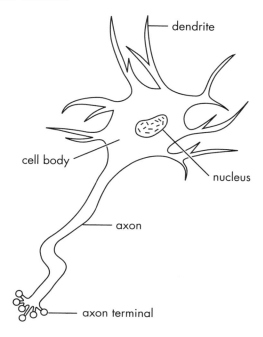

Figure 5.2 The synapse

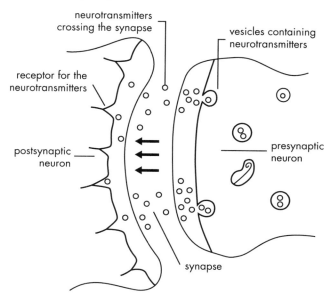

ALZHEIMER'S DISEASE

Alzheimer's disease is the most common type of dementia, accounting for about 50 to 60 per cent of cases. It is named after the German neurologist Alois Alzheimer, who first described the neuropathology (brain pathology) in a famous lecture in 1906. The subject was a woman with symptoms of hallucinations, disorientation and memory loss that progressed over some years until her death at the age of 55 years. Alzheimer identified the two major abnormalities in the brain that characterise the disease— senile plaques and neurofibrillary tangles in the cortex of the brain. His senior colleague, Emil Kraepelin, who is regarded as one of the founding figures of modern psychiatry, named the disease after Alzheimer.

For the next 60 or 70 years Alzheimer's disease was considered to be a rare condition that caused pre-senile dementia in people under the age of 65 years. Senile dementia, which developed in late life, was regarded as a separate disorder. It was considered either as a normal part of the ageing process (senescence) or as due to arteriosclerotic changes (hardening of the arteries) in cerebral blood vessels. However, research in Newcastle upon Tyne in the United Kingdom, published in the early 1970s, demonstrated that senile dementia and Alzheimer's disease were the same condition.[2] This has led to the explosion of research over the last 30 years.

As described in detail in Chapter 4, Alzheimer's disease is a gradually progressive disorder with a course of six to twelve years, though there have been people who have died within twelve months and others who have survived for 20 years. Symptoms may be present for several years before diagnosis. There is evidence that brain abnormalities are present for at least 30 years before symptoms become apparent, so the true course of the disease may be closer to 50 years. Clearly, this provides an opportunity for interventions that could be applied before symptoms are apparent—providing that accurate identification of non-symptomatic Alzheimer's disease were possible through a diagnostic test of blood, urine or cerebrospinal fluid (CSF). Such tests are otherwise known as 'peripheral biomarkers' of Alzheimer's disease because they do not involve direct testing of the central nervous system. There are already some exciting prospects on the horizon, which are considered in Chapter 13.

Our understanding about what happens to the brain in Alzheimer's disease has increased dramatically in recent years, even if the precise reasons that the disease processes commence are not fully understood. The genetic influences on its development are fully covered in Chapter 3 and are not repeated here.

As an overview, the Alzheimer's disease process initially destroys nerve cells in parts of the brain that control memory, including the hippocampus and related structures. With damage to the hippocampus, short-term memory fails, impacting upon the person's daily function. Later the brain cortex, particularly the areas responsible for language and reasoning, becomes affected. Eventually, many other areas of the brain are involved and they atrophy (shrink) and lose function.[3]

Senile (amyloid) plaques and the amyloid cascade hypothesis

As mentioned earlier, Alzheimer was the first to describe senile plaques. These consist of largely insoluble deposits of a type of protein known as beta-amyloid protein, and hence are sometimes called amyloid plaques. Beta-amyloid protein is derived from a larger protein called amyloid precursor protein (APP). The beta-amyloid aggregates (clumps) together, mixed with debris from neurons (nerve cells) and other cells, to form the plaques. Although they can be found in normal older people, in Alzheimer's disease the plaques are predominantly found in areas of the brain used for memory and other cognitive functions—the hippocampus, medial temporal lobe and parietal lobe. Plaques are not likely to be the cause of the dementia. They are more likely to be a by-product of the disease process. Amyloid production, however, is central to the disease process.

John Hardy proposed the amyloid cascade hypothesis in the early 1990s after the discovery of mutations on the APP gene that were found to be associated with a rare form of early onset Alzheimer's disease. In essence, the amyloid cascade hypothesis states that amyloid deposits in Alzheimer's disease result from a number of genetic or environmental insults and lead to the degeneration of nerve cells that results in dementia. As beta-amyloid is derived from APP, a large protein with an unknown function found throughout the brain, understanding the process by which it is produced from APP is of critical importance as it may provide a target for future treatments. APP is metabolised (broken down) in two distinct ways, only one of which results in the formation of beta-amyloid. Both are normal processes, thus explaining why some plaques are found in normal people.[4]

In the rare early onset Alzheimer's disease, there is over-production of beta-amyloid and increased plaque formation. In late onset Alzheimer's disease, while there is normal production of beta-amyloid, there is a failure to degrade it which results in plaque formation. This implies that two basic therapeutic approaches could be applied—firstly, inhibit the production of beta-amyloid; secondly, facilitate the degradation of beta-amyloid. However, it is unclear whether removal of beta-amyloid plaques will result in any improvement in mental function. As described in Chapter 13, research into these approaches is currently underway.

How does amyloid cause neurodegeneration?

In describing the disease process, so far I have made little mention of damage to nerve cells, which clearly has to occur for dementia to develop. Alzheimer's disease is characterised by abnormal cell death of vulnerable nerve cells in regions of the brain that are essential to normal cognitive function. It is this cell death that results in the brain atrophy, detectable on brain scans, so charac-teristic of the disease. Amyloid may increase 'programmed cell death' in the brain, an essentially normal process that helps weed out unnecessary or diseased cells, but which in the adult brain may result in irreversible loss of brain cells and function. It may open up calcium channels into the neuron allowing uncontrolled amounts of calcium to kill the cell.[5] Another possibility, suggested by Colin Masters from Melbourne University, is that it is the small amount of *soluble* amyloid present (in contrast to the *insoluble* amyloid in plaques) that may be associated with damage to cells.[6]

Neurofibrillary tangles and tau protein

The second feature of Alzheimer's disease as originally described by Alzheimer is the neurofibrillary tangle. Neurofibrillary tangles (NFTs) are composed of a protein called tau. They are found in other degenerative disorders such as frontotemporal dementia. In contrast to plaques, the number of NFTs found in the brain and their anatomical localisation is strongly associated with the severity of dementia. Further, the NFTs are contained within the nerve cells and there is strong evidence to show that their presence heralds cell death. Thus there is strong circumstantial evidence that NFTs are essential components of the process that results in dementia. Tau protein normally stabilises the micro-tubules in the neuron which are essential for the fast transport of microscopic components through the nerve cell. Damage to the microtubules results in loss of function of the neuron. In Alzheimer's disease, tau protein loses its ability to promote micro-tubule assembly and forms into NFTs.[7]

This is a controversial area and for many years there have been two schools of thought as to whether amyloid deposition or NFTs are the fundamental cause of Alzheimer's disease. (Humorists have labelled the two schools as BAPtists, for Beta-Amyloid Protein, and TAUists.) Certainly, most evidence points to beta-amyloid as being the initial abnormality, with NFT formation coming later. As in most complex systems, however, it is likely that both are critical to the disease process.

Neurotransmitters

Neurons communicate with each other by secreting chemicals known as neurotransmitters that bridge the microscopic gap between nerve cells at a point called the synapse (see Figure 5.2). This is a complicated process that involves numerous steps, each of which may either inhibit or enhance the communication. There are numerous neurotransmitters in the brain, including serotonin, noradrenaline, dopamine and acetylcholine. In Alzheimer's disease, it has long been established that the neurons secreting acetylcholine are the major ones affected by the disease. Acetylcholine (cholinergic) pathways are critically important for normal memory function. It is not surprising that from the time of the initial recognition of the role of acetylcholine in Alzheimer's disease treatments to overcome the deficiency were trialled. After considerable early disappointment, when efforts to directly boost the level of acetylcholine in the brain were ineffec-tive, agents that indirectly boost the level of acetylcholine in the synapse by reducing its breakdown have been effective. These treatments are described in more detail in Chapter 7.

Many other neurotransmitters are affected in Alzheimer's disease, including glutamate, which has an effect on learning, serotonin, which is important for mood, and GABA, which has a role in anxiety and aggression. Neurotransmitters also interact, so that release of one may have a modulating effect on another. An important issue to appreciate is that changes in neurotransmission in Alzheimer's disease only occur after there has been significant cell death. Acetylcholine deficiency is a result of the disease process, not a cause, thus treatments that enhance the amount of acetylcholine in the brain are unlikely to alter the underlying disease process in a major way.[8]

In summary, Alzheimer's disease is an age-related neurodegenerative disorder involving the clumping together of abnormal beta-amyloid and tau proteins in the brain over many years. This eventually results in a gradually progressive dementia due to neuronal dysfunction and cell death, particularly in the hippocampus, medial, temporal and parietal lobes of the brain. Although numerous risk factors have been identified, as outlined in Chapters 2 and 3, most determine when the disease becomes symptomatic rather than being causal factors.

Vascular dementia

Some people believe that vascular dementia has been the 'forgotten' dementia, because of the degree of media attention given to Alzheimer's disease. Further, the relative lack of research interest into treatments means that currently no memory-enhancing drugs approved for vascular dementia are available in Australia. Yet vascular dementia is the second most common type of dementia in Australia, accounting for 15 to 20 per cent of cases, while perhaps 25 per cent of Alzheimer cases also have some vascular changes in the brain. It is more common in men than women in the general population, and in both men and women of Chinese and Japanese descent. Vascular dementia is diagnosed when disease affecting blood vessels in the brain (cerebrovascular disease) is judged to be causal to the dementia. In contrast to Alzheimer's disease, a variety of processes is responsible for the dementia, and thus there is a wide range of clinical presentations.

Historically, vascular dementia has been described under a number of different terms. In the nineteenth century, 'arteriosclerotic dementia' was a term commonly used for what today would be mainly diagnosed as Alzheimer's disease. It was also recognised that apoplexy (stroke) often resulted in permanent changes in mental function, when the term 'post-apoplectic dementia' was used. Following the better delineation of Alzheimer's disease, Hachinski in 1974 coined the term 'multi-infarct dementia' to describe the dementia that results from multiple cerebral infarcts (strokes). As there are forms of dementia caused by cerebrovascular disease that are not due to multiple infarcts, the term 'vascular dementia' was introduced in the 1990s as an umbrella term.[9]

Vascular dementia may result from single or multiple causes. The main causes are haemodynamic (blood flow to the brain) disorders (for example, strokes), thromboembolism (small blood clots originating mainly from the carotid artery or heart that block small blood vessels in the brain), small blood vessel disease in the brain (which results in a gradual reduction in blood supply to the brain), and haemorrhage (bleeding) into or around the brain (subarachnoid, intracerebral or subdural). Dementia following stroke is particularly common, occurring in one-quarter to one-third of stroke victims, particularly when certain strategic areas of the brain are affected, such as the frontal subcortical regions. Some researchers also hypothesise that stroke victims who develop dementia have early features of Alzheimer's disease that were not severe enough to cause symptoms before the stroke, but that reduce the brain reserve and leave the person vulnerable to the effects of the stroke. Prognosis is often poor, as the risk of further stroke is high.[10]

Due to this range of causal disorders, in comparison with Alzheimer's disease the onset of symptoms in vascular dementia is quite variable. Some symptoms may follow a sudden stroke; in other cases there may be a gradually progressive pattern with some fluctuation; in yet others there is the classic stepwise deterioration, in which a sudden decline is followed by a period of stability before another sudden decline, and so on. To further complicate matters, some cases of vascular dementia are clinically almost indistinguishable from Alzheimer's disease, with gradual onset of slowly progressive cognitive impairment.

The Hachinski Scale was developed to help clinicians distinguish vascular dementia from Alzheimer's disease on clinical grounds. The items on the scale indicate clinical features that are more likely to occur in vascular dementia than in Alzheimer's disease. These include hypertension (high blood pressure), depression, focal neurological symptoms (for example, limb paresis or weakness) or signs (for example, abnormal reflexes), sudden onset and stepwise decline. Diagnosis of vascular dementia is aided by the demonstration of lesions caused by vascular disease on CT or MRI scans; in the absence of such findings, however, accurate differentiation from Alzheimer's disease can be difficult if there has been an 'Alzheimer-type' onset. This difficulty is reflected in the lack of consensus between four internationally recognised sets of clinical diagnostic criteria for vascular dementia. Some clinicians tend to label all difficult to diagnose cases as 'mixed dementia', others as Alzheimer's disease. This is probably the major source of diagnostic inaccuracy in dementia assessment.[11]

Because of this variety of pathologies responsible for vascular dementia, the clinical course of the disease is highly variable, though on the whole there is a worse prognosis than for Alzheimer's disease. This may be due to the fact that people with vascular dementia are more likely to have serious cardiovascular disorders and other associated conditions, including diabetes, hypertension, peripheral vascular disease and smoking-related disorders. Consequently, the general medical management of the person with vascular dementia is of much greater importance than in Alzheimer's disease. Control of hypertension and diabetes, low dose aspirin to reduce blood clotting, cessation of smoking, reduction of cholesterol, adequate exercise, moderate alcohol intake, weight control, stress management and low fat/low salt diets are all possible interventions.

DEMENTIA WITH LEWY BODIES

Dementia with Lewy bodies (DLB) has only been recognised as a distinct entity over the last decade. It is estimated to account for between 10 and 20 per cent of dementia cases. It tends to occur in the age range of 50 to 85 years, and is slightly more common in males. The mean duration of the disease is four and a half years, though it ranges from one to 20 years. There is significant overlap with Alzheimer's disease, with many patients having both disorders; indeed, for many years what is now known as DLB was thought to be a clinical subtype of Alzheimer's disease.

This is one of the reasons for the delineation of the disorder being so recent. Consensus guidelines for diagnosis only appeared in 1996.[12]

The clinical features of DLB are quite striking. Onset of the disorder tends to be relatively sudden in comparison with Alzheimer's disease. The progressive cognitive decline is featured by poor attention and visuospatial function (ability of the brain to integrate visual and spatial information) but relatively intact memory. Cognition tends to fluctuate to the extent that the patient may appear to be in an acute confusional state; frequently, however, extensive hospital investigation fails to identify a cause. At other times fluctuating cognition may simply be mistaken for daytime tiredness. Visual hallucinations are often prominent early in the course of the illness and usually involve animals or people, sometimes frightening but often not. Features of parkinsonism with muscular rigidity, tremors and slowed movements are common, but characteristically these develop alongside the cognitive changes. When Parkinson's disease has been present for a year or more before the dementia, it is more correctly diagnosed as Parkinson's disease dementia. Recurrent falls, faints that are often misdiagnosed as transient ischaemic attacks (TIAs), depression and sensitivity to antipsychotic medication (often prescribed for the hallucinations) are supportive diagnostic features.[13]

Lewy bodies are found in neurons and contain the protein alpha-synuclein, which interferes with neuronal function. Lewy, who worked in the same laboratory as Alzheimer, first described them in 1912. They have long been recognised as being the main brain abnormality of Parkinson's disease. Although regularly noted to be present in the cortical areas of brains of Alzheimer patients, until the early 1990s this was thought to be an incidental finding as the number present seemed insufficient to cause brain damage.

At about this time new laboratory techniques resulted in the Lewy bodies being more easily seen under the microscope. Suddenly, researchers in Newcastle upon Tyne and San Diego in particular became aware that Lewy bodies were present in large amounts in the brains of up to 36 per cent of Alzheimer patients. Because Lewy bodies are so pale, they had been very difficult to see in cerebral white matter with the standard stains used for the previous century. This quickly led to a re-evaluation of the clinical syndrome. Similar to Alzheimer's disease, there is a marked deficit in acetylcholine in the brain but there are also deficits of the neurotransmitter dopamine. The cholinergic deficits mean that the cholinesterase-inhibitor drugs primarily designed for Alzheimer's disease are also beneficial in DLB, with some experience suggesting a better response than found in Alzheimer's disease.[14]

FRONTOTEMPORAL DEMENTIA

Frontotemporal dementia is a term used to describe a group of neurodegenerative disorders that includes Pick's disease. It accounts for approximately 10 per cent of dementia cases and is particularly common in younger age groups, usually developing between the ages of 35 and 75 years, with no gender differences. Frontotemporal dementia primarily affects the frontal and anterior temporal lobes of the brain. These areas control what are described as 'executive functions'—reasoning, judgement, insight, personality, social behaviour, speech, language and certain aspects of memory. Frontotemporal dementia runs a course of between two and ten years after diagnosis.

In 20 to 40 per cent of cases there is a family history of dementia, so it seems that there is a strong genetic component in the disease. In 1998 it was discovered that a mutation in the tau gene linked to chromosome 17 causes a form of frontotemporal dementia called 'frontotemporal dementia with parkinsonism'. One major similarity to Alzheimer's disease is the characteristic accumulation of abnormal tau protein inside nerve cells in neurofibrillary tangles (NFTs), disrupting normal nerve cell processes and ultimately leading to cell death. Other changes include a progressive loss of nerve cells in the frontal and temporal regions of the brain, gliosis (nerve tissue scarring) and vacuolation, a process in which 'holes' form in the outer layer of the brain. In Pick's disease, characteristic Pick bodies are found in neurons.

Frontotemporal dementia has an insidious onset. Behaviour and personality change, such as irritability, apathy, inappropriate sexual behaviour, compulsive behaviours and loss of awareness or concern about behaviour change, are the most frequent clinical features at presentation. In other cases language impairment may be the initial clinical feature, with a lack of spontaneous speech, often interpreted by family members as being due to disinterest or depression. Another type of speech impairment involves stuttering with frequent paraphasic errors where the wrong word is used (for example, saying that a comb is a brush), the use of non-grammatical speech and stereotypical speech where the same words, phrases or themes are repeated. The initial clinical features depend on the side of the brain primarily damaged—language deficits predominate when the left side is primarily affected; behavioural problems develop more with right-sided disease. With behavioural and personality changes it can be some years before it becomes apparent that there may be an underlying brain disorder. This is particularly the case in a younger person, where problems may initially be attributed to such diverse issues as work stress, depression, alcohol or drug abuse, marital disharmony or the menopause. Eventually memory and language impairment become more obvious. People with frontotemporal dementia may also develop motor difficulties like those seen in Parkinson's disease. These include muscle rigidity, lack of balance and stiffness of movement, but not the limb tremors at rest that are characteristic of Parkinson's.

The diagnostic assessment of people with suspected fronto-temporal dementia usually requires a neuropsychological evaluation as part of the dementia work-up, as many of the standard cognitive tests used in routine dementia assessment are relatively insensitive to impaired frontal lobe function. At times even the initial neuropsychological evaluation will be equivocal, and repeat testing six to twelve months later may be necessary. One major difference between frontotemporal dementia and Alzheimer's disease is that people with frontotemporal dementia do not suffer as much memory loss, tend to know where they are, and are able to recall information about the past and present. Even in the late stages, people with frontotemporal dementia, unlike those with Alzheimer's disease, are able to negotiate their surroundings and remain well oriented.[15]

Currently there are no specific treatments available that can slow or stop the disease process. Other general treatments for some of the symptoms and behaviours are covered in Chapter 7.

OTHER NEURODEGENERATIVE CAUSES OF DEMENTIA

Parkinson's disease characteristically presents with tremors, slowing of limb movements and increased muscle tone or stiffness. A shuffling style of walking with a stooped posture and lack of arm swing is common. Parkinson's disease that develops in late life has a high risk of progressing to dementia, with features that are often similar to dementia with Lewy bodies.

A range of other less common neurodegenerative disorders also cause dementia.

Corticobasal degeneration and *progressive supranuclear palsy* are related to frontotemporal dementia inasmuch as they are caused by tau protein aggregation in neurons. Corticobasal degeneration has symptoms that often appear to be a mix of Parkinson's and Alzheimer's disease. Progressive supranuclear palsy, the disease from which the English comedian Dudley Moore died, mainly involves the brain stem and areas known as the basal ganglia. The clinical features include those of Parkinson's disease: instability when standing and walking (the sufferer may appear 'intoxicated' and have falls), and difficulties in looking upwards with the eyes.[16]

Creutzfeldt-Jakob disease (CJD) is a prion disease. Prions are small glycoproteins with infectious qualities that cause amyloid formation and nerve degeneration. CJD is characterised by a rapidly progressive dementia (death usually occurs within two years) with features of myoclonus (muscular jerks), unsteadiness of gait and neurological features implying involvement of cortical and subcortical structures of the brain. Although most attention has been given in the popular press to infectious forms, particularly that associated with bovine spongiform encephalopathy (BSE or mad cow disease), there is also a very rare inherited form that accounts for between 5 and 10 per cent of cases. A mutation on the PRNP gene accounts for 70 per cent of the inherited form of CJD worldwide.[17]

Huntington's disease is a genetic disorder with abnormalities on chromosome 4. All carriers of the gene will get the disease and children of carriers have a 50 per cent chance of getting it. It is a neurodegenerative disorder characterised by abnormal involuntary movements of the body (choreiform movements), personality change, and psychiatric problems that usually predate the dementing process. It usually has an age of onset between 30 and

45 years, but cases outside this age range also occur. Sporadic cases without a known family history can occur.[18]

Familial British dementia (FBD) is a rare disease characterised by progressive dementia, paralysis and loss of balance. It usually occurs around age 40 to 50. Similar to Alzheimer's disease, FBD patients have amyloid deposition associated with blood vessels and NFTs. It is due to a defect in the gene called BRI, which is located on chromosome 13. A close variant of the disorder was recently found in a small Danish population.[19]

OTHER DEMENTIAS

Some of the other less common types of dementia are potentially reversible, and are the focus of investigations during dementia assessment as described in Chapter 6. These include neurosyphilis (the late stage of untreated syphilis that may occur many years after the initial venereal infection), disorders of the thyroid gland, deficiencies of vitamin B_{12} and folic acid, chronic drug intoxication, chronic meningitis, cerebral vasculitis due to auto-immune disorders such as temporal arteritis and various metabolic disorders.

Normal pressure hydrocephalus is a condition in which an intermittent blockage of the flow of cerebrospinal fluid (CSF) around the brain can result in marked dilatation of the cerebral ventricles (cistern-like structures inside the brain) through build-up of the CSF and subsequent compression and death of brain tissue. The early symptoms are gait disturbances, incontinence of urine and confusion, usually developing over a few months. It tends to occur in younger people (most commonly 40 to 70 years of age) and is predisposed by a history of meningitis, subarachnoid haemorrhage, head trauma or cerebral tumours, although in nearly 50 per cent of cases there is no known cause. After it was first described in the 1960s, many dementia patients who had a gait disturbance and urinary incontinence, and were found to have large cerebral ventricles on brain scan, had neurosurgery in which a shunt was placed into the brain to drain away the excess CSF. Approximately 50 per cent of patients improved, usually those whose symptoms had developed in the previous few months, had a known cause for the condition and did not have signs of brain atrophy on scans. It became clear, however, that many of those operated upon, particularly those with dementia symptoms for over six months and without any other obvious cause for the dilatation of the cerebral ventricles, did not have normal pressure hydrocephalus. Indeed, they were mainly Alzheimer patients. Furthermore, there were frequent surgical complications, especially infections of the implanted shunts that necessitated repeated procedures.[20] Normal pressure hydrocephalus is infrequently diagnosed now, but new interest has been expressed in the last year about the use of shunts as a treatment for Alzheimer's disease (see Chapter 13).

Alcoholic dementia is a somewhat controversial diagnosis. It is clear that alcohol abuse and associated thiamine deficiency can cause severe brain damage known as Wernicke-Korsakoff disorder, which has profound chronic short-term memory impairment (see Chapter 6) without other features of dementia. In autopsy studies of the brains of people diagnosed with alcoholic dementia, no specific abnormality in the brain has been identified, with most cases being found to have either vascular dementia or Alzheimer's disease. Still, it remains a diagnosis that is frequently used in areas of Australia with high rates of alcohol abuse.

Head injuries that cause dementia are usually very severe, and it may be some months before sufficient recovery from the acute confusion has occurred to determine what deficits remain. One characteristic of this form of dementia is that improvement may continue for some years after the injury. In those who recover, a delayed onset of dementia may occur some years later, as indicated by head injury being a risk factor for Alzheimer's disease.

Brain tumours are discovered quite frequently in dementia investigation. Most are small, inconsequential, benign meningiomas that have little effect and don't require treatment. Some are large enough and located at a site to warrant surgical removal. In my experience this rarely results in cognitive improvement, but may prevent further decline. Occasionally malignant tumours such as gliomas may cause dementia, and here the prognosis is very poor.

HIV/AIDS dementia complex occurs in up to 15 per cent of HIV-infected adults. In over 90 per cent of cases it develops in the last year of life. Unlike other AIDS-defining illnesses, the standard highly active antiretroviral therapy has not had much impact on the development of the illness, possibly due to poor central nervous system penetration. Therapy has been limited by an incomplete understanding of how the AIDS dementia complex occurs. There is also an absence of large, adequate and well-controlled clinical trials using agents that protect nerve cells or agents with disease-modifying potential. In general, people with AIDS dementia complex have little involvement with mainstream dementia services. This is in part due to their average age of around 35 years.[21]

SUMMARY

Apart from vascular dementia, most common types of dementia, including Alzheimer's disease, are caused by the gradual abnormal accumulation of toxic proteins in the brain that results in neuro-degeneration, in turn resulting in impaired neuronal function and cell death.

CHAPTER 6

DEMENTIA ASSESSMENT

'AM I GETTING DEMENTIA?' Some people ask this question because they have noticed a change in their memory. There are many reasons for older people acquiring symptoms that may raise fears within themselves, in their families, their friends or their doctors about the possibility that they are developing dementia. Subjective concerns about cognitive performance are most frequently due to awareness of normal age-related cognitive change, anxiety, depression and various medical problems such as thyroid underactivity.

> Carmel had always been a 'worrier'; now, at the age of 70 she was concerned that her memory was failing. She complained to her doctor that she kept forgetting the reason that she had gone from one room to another in her home, but admitted that after some minutes it would usually come back to her. She couldn't recall the details of conversations she had with her husband and friends, though she remembered having the conversations. And, of course, she could never remember people's names and that was so embarrassing! Recently, she had felt under some stress. Her older daughter had divorced, her husband had suffered a heart attack though was now well, and a good friend had died.

It is important to get a basic check-up with your doctor if you are in this situation, as there may be a simple explanation for what you have noticed which will respond to treatment. If there is no simple explanation, a dementia assessment may be called for. This assessment aims to determine the cause of the worrying symptoms and to recommend appropriate management.

WHAT IS DEMENTIA ASSESSMENT?

The precise components of the assessment process for dementia will vary according to the nature of the presenting symptoms and the centre where it is undertaken, but there are a number of basic principles. As noted in Chapter 4, early symptoms of dementia may be subtle and equivocal. In this circumstance, the initial focus will be to determine whether or not the problem is caused by dementia or some other condition. Where people present for assessment with symptoms of well-established dementia, the main focus will be on establishing the type of dementia. In either circumstance, dementia assessment includes gathering all aspects of information about a person that will enable an accurate identification of the symptoms—that is, description of behaviours, identification of psychosocial issues, measurement of functional capacity and determination of relevant medical conditions (which will certainly include a range of diagnostic investigations). An adequate assessment requires the involvement of the person's spouse, children, siblings, friends and occasionally parents to corroborate information, to provide additional details from an observer perspective and usually to allow an assessment of their needs as carers or potential carers.[1]

WHO SHOULD PERFORM THE ASSESSMENT?

Initial assessment—screening

A range of assessment options is available in most places. Ideally, the person's general practitioner should undertake the initial assessment, but other possibilities include the local Aged Care Assessment Team or, if the person is hospitalised for some reason, hospital doctors. In each of these settings, it is commonplace these days for a routine screening examination to be performed on all elderly patients, especially those aged over 75.

Screening involves a brief examination of mental function to determine whether there are signs of possible dementia or another mental and/or physical disorder. Most general practitioners have been taught how to use at least one of a number of screening tests for cognitive function that take five to ten minutes to complete. Examples include the Abbreviated Mental Test Score

(AMTS), the seven-minute screen (7MS), the Mini-Mental State Examination (MMSE) and GP-COG. Each of these tests has in common questions that check the person's orientation, immediate memory and short-term memory in a standardised fashion. For example, 'what day of the week is it?' is included in most tests to check orientation in time, while recalling either a set of words or a name and address both immediately and after about three minutes is used to check memory function. Other cognitive functions are covered to varying degrees in the different tests.

The tests are standardised, so the scores obtained give an indication as to whether there is likely to be a significant impairment of cognitive function requiring a more substantial examination. On the MMSE the 'cut-off' score is 24 out of 30; on the AMTS it is 7 out of 10. This doesn't mean that a score below the cut-off scores equates with dementia. A person who is severely depressed or suffering from a severe infection may score well below the cut-off when unwell but well above when recovered. Other factors that may lower scores include poor education, poor hearing, limited English language skills, lifelong developmental delay and severe psychiatric disorders such as schizophrenia.

Similarly, some people with early dementia will score above the cut-off. This is more likely to happen with an intelligent person who may have declined from their pre-morbid level of cognitive function, but not sufficiently to be detected by the screen. Thus, to improve the chances of detecting a clinically significant problem, it is advisable for the GP to obtain collateral information from the person's partner, friends or family. The advantage of the GP-COG (see Table 6.1), developed in Australia by Professor Henry Brodaty and colleagues in Sydney, is that it includes some questions to elicit such information as part of the standardised scale. Even if the screening test was above the cut-off score, further assessment would be warranted if informants had noticed a decline, particularly if the score was just above the cut-off or points had been lost on the short-term memory task.[2]

This initial assessment, when allied with a general check-up, should identify most persons likely to have early dementia and who require a more thorough examination. Others will have been found to be anxious, depressed or have some other medical problem, as described later, that is responsible for the symptoms. This group should have these problems treated and have their

Table 6.1 GP-COG (Brodaty et al., 2002)

Patient examination

Name and address for subsequent recall test

1. *I am going to give you a name and address. After I have said it, I want you to repeat it. Remember this name and address because I am going to ask you to tell it to me again in a few minutes: John Brown, 42 West Street, Kensington* (allow 4 attempts—this is not scored)

Time orientation

2. *What is the date?* (exact only = 1 point)

Clock drawing—use a page with a printed circle

3. *Please mark in all the numbers to indicate the hours of a clock* (correct spacing required = 1 point)

4. *Please mark in hands to show 10 minutes past 11 o'clock* (11.10 = 1 point)

Information

5. *Can you tell me something that happened in the news recently?* (recently = past week = 1 point if reasonable detail)

Memory recall

6. *What was the name and address I asked you to remember?* (5 points— one each for 'John', 'Brown', '42', 'West' and 'Kensington')

Score of 9—normal, no further testing

Scores of 5–8—proceed to informant interview

Scores of 0–4—abnormal, doesn't require informant interview

Informant interview

Ask the informant:

Compared to a few years ago:

Does the patient have more trouble remembering things that have happened recently? (No = 1)

Does he or she have more trouble recalling conversations a few days later? (No = 1)

When speaking, does the patient have more difficulty in finding the right word or tend to use the wrong words more often? (No = 1)

Is the patient less able to manage money and financial affairs (e.g. paying bills, budgeting)? (No = 1)

Is the patient less able to manage his or her medication independently? (No = 1)

Does the patient need more assistance with transport (either private or public)? (No = 1)

Scores of 4–6—normal

Scores of 0–3—cognitive impairment

cognition reviewed when they have fully recovered. A third group has symptoms that do not appear to be significant—they score above the cut-offs on the screening tests and their informants haven't noticed much change. In most cases it would be reasonable to take a 'wait-and-see' approach by reviewing the situation every six months. However, if either the general practitioner or the patient were uneasy with this, it would be wise to seek a specialist opinion.

Definitive assessment

A definitive assessment should contain a number of components, as listed in Table 6.2.

Table 6.2 Domains of definitive dementia assessment

- Full history, full mental state examination (including cognitive assessment with a reliable standardised scale) and physical examination of person with cognitive problems by an appropriately trained medical practitioner.
- Collateral history from support person (partner, sibling, child, friend) to obtain a description of the cognitive, behavioural and functional changes in addition to medical history.
- Identification of psychosocial issues including any potential relationship difficulties between the dementing person and their main supports, carer concerns and stress, financial circumstances, knowledge/fears about dementia.
- Measurement of functional capacity including work, driving, financial competency (power of attorney, will).
- Appropriate laboratory, radiological and other investigations as required to establish the correct diagnosis.
- These combine:
  to construct a prioritised problem list;
  to determine the cause of the cognitive change;
  to devise a management plan with the patient and their supporters that includes:
  - explanation of the diagnosis or further action required to determine the diagnosis
  - dementia education and information about appropriate services including the Alzheimer's Association
  - treatment options
  - planning for the future—wills, financial management, driving competency
  - answering any questions about the diagnosis
  - follow-up arrangements

Once it has been determined that a more thorough assessment is required, this almost certainly means an examination by a medical specialist—psychiatrist, neurologist or geriatrician, depending on local availability and the type of presenting symptoms. For example, a person who is depressed with memory loss may be better off seeing a psychiatrist, either an old age psychiatrist (psychogeriatrician) or a neuropsychiatrist. An aged person with multiple medical problems and confusion might best see a geriatrician. Neurologists might be the most appropriate specialists to see younger persons with cognitive impairment, persons with rapidly progressive cognitive change, or persons with other neurological symptoms such as gait problems. This does not necessarily mean an immediate referral. Many GPs will quite appropriately do a more detailed examination and undertake the routine investigations described in Table 6.3 before referral. Frequently a GP will determine the correct diagnosis but most will prefer to have this confirmed by a specialist, particularly now that the Pharmaceutical Benefit Scheme (PBS) regulations for prescribing cholinesterase inhibitor drugs for Alzheimer's disease demand specialist confirmation.

Memory clinics are another option in many parts of Australia. These are mainly based in the public health system in hospitals and community centres. In Victoria they have been based in aged care services and called Cognitive Dementia and Memory Services (CDAMS) and since 1997 have been developed in a network throughout the State in order to improve dementia assessment and management. The advantages of memory clinics are that they are thorough, specialise in dementia assessment and are usually multidisciplinary. Most routinely involve neuropsychologists for a more detailed cognitive assessment, social workers to assess the family circumstances, occupational therapists to determine the person's level of function, and community nurses, in addition to one or more of the medical specialists previously mentioned (see Table 6.4). Usually there is an assessment protocol that involves examination by the various health professionals over a number of sessions spread over a few weeks. The protocol includes the various diagnostic investigations required to make an accurate dementia diagnosis. The final diagnosis and management recommendations are often determined by consensus opinion from the various team members.

Table 6.3 Dementia investigations

Routine investigations	Reason(s) for the investigation
Full blood count	To exclude anaemia, infections
Urea, creatinine and electrolytes	To exclude kidney and metabolic disorders
Calcium	To exclude high calcium, e.g. due to tumours
Liver function tests	To exclude liver failure, liver tumours
Serum vitamin B_{12} and red blood cell folate	To exclude deficiency states, pernicious anaemia
Erythrocyte sedimentation rate (ESR)	Often abnormal in inflammatory conditions such as vasculitis and infections
Thyroid function tests	To exclude overactive and underactive thyroid
Brain CT scan	To exclude strokes, tumours, subdural haematomas and hydrocephalus, and to determine whether atrophy is present
Chest X-ray	To exclude tumours and infections

Investigations required when clinically indicated	Reason(s) for the investigation
Neuropsychological examination	To distinguish mild cognitive impairment from early dementia and to assist in diagnosing the type of dementia
Brain MRI scan	To exclude vasculitis or encephalopathy and to obtain higher resolution brain images
Electrocardiogram (ECG) and Holter monitor	To exclude cardiac causes of vascular dementia
Carotid dopplers	To exclude carotid artery disease as a cause of vascular dementia
Echocardiogram	To exclude cardiac causes of vascular dementia
Fasting blood sugar level	To exclude diabetes mellitus
Syphilis serology	To exclude syphilis infection
Microurine	To exclude urinary tract infections and renal disease
Electroencephalogram (EEG)	To exclude epilepsy and encephalopathy
Lumbar puncture	To exclude meningitis or encephalitis
SPECT or PET scan	To assist in the diagnosis of early Alzheimer's disease and vascular dementia
Human immunodeficiency virus (HIV) screen	To exclude HIV/AIDS-related disorder
Immunological screen	To exclude vasculitis due to auto-immune disorders
Genetic screening	For those at risk of Huntington's disease, familial forms of Alzheimer's disease or frontotemporal dementia

Table 6.4 Components of multidisciplinary dementia assessment

Medical assessment

This involves a full medical history, mental state examination and full physical examination. The history is usually obtained from both the dementing person and the primary informant to enable a more accurate understanding of the problems. The mental state examination explores both cognitive and psychological functioning to determine the extent of cognitive deficits and whether there is a psychiatric disorder, especially depression, present. Often a depression scale is used. The physical examination focuses mainly on the neurological system.

Neuropsychological assessment

This is a two to three hour assessment performed by a trained neuropsychologist using a battery of standardised tests to evaluate cognitive functions in different parts of the brain. Test scores are compared with population norms; some tests are designed to enable an estimation of function before the onset of disease. They are particularly useful in quantifying memory impairment and in determining the pattern of cognitive deficits that may help in determining the type of dementia. Where deficits are mild or equivocal, repeat testing in six to twelve months may elicit changes not detected by other assessments. Neuropsychologists are usually only available in major centres.

Social work assessment

There are two basic strands to this assessment. One focuses on the social function and support network of the dementing person and attempts to determine whether any additional social supports are required. The other focuses on the dementing person's family and other carers, assessing their level of stress and how well they are coping. In some centres, this latter assessment may be linked with carer support groups. The social worker will often be responsible for arranging whatever community services are determined to be necessary.

Occupational therapy assessment

This assessment is usually carried out in the dementing person's home. It aims to determine their functional capacity by assessing their ability to perform various activities of daily living. In those with mild cognitive impairments, the assessment concentrates on higher order activities such

continues . . .

Table 6.4 Components of multidisciplinary dementia assessment (continued)

as financial management, meal preparation, telephone use and organisational skills. Driving assessments are often undertaken as a separate task. Where there are more severe deficits, more basic skills such as dressing, bathing and toileting are covered. An assessment of the home for basic safety is also done—for example, if the person has a history of falls, recommendations might be made about the installation of rails.

Nursing assessment
In many centres, community nurses perform a combination of cognitive screening, social work and occupational therapy-style assessments. This is especially the case where the community nurse is part of an aged care assessment team. Medication management is a common issue that requires assessment in those who live alone.

Memory clinics may not be suitable for assessing all cases of dementia. They are probably most useful in suspected early dementia and where there are no major associated medical or psychological problems. A geriatrician and the aged care assessment team may better assess frail older people, and those with more severe cognitive impairment of long standing, in the person's home. Similarly, aged care mental health services would be better for assessing depressed or psychotic persons with suspected dementia. Assessments by these other services will include many of the multidisciplinary assessments that take place in memory clinics, but are more likely to be tailored to the individual case. For example, many people with mild dementia, and most with moderate–severe dementia, will not require a neuropsychological examination.

It is not essential that all these assessments be undertaken in every case during the initial assessment process. For example, in very mild dementia it may not be necessary to have an occupational therapy assessment, as there are few relevant deficits. Also, many doctors give sufficient time to family members to talk over their concerns; if they are coping without significant problems, a social work assessment may not be required. The other assessments can be undertaken at a later date if the situation changes.

WHAT ELSE MAY BE CAUSING MEMORY CHANGES?
THE DIFFERENTIAL DIAGNOSIS OF DEMENTIA

Throughout the assessment process, the aim is to eliminate any other condition as the cause of the person's cognitive impairment before determining the type of dementia. The main conditions that need to be excluded are described here.

Depression

In Chapter 4, I demonstrated how depression might be the forerunner of dementia. There are also situations where depression may mimic dementia. After the age of 40, most people who become clinically depressed are likely to have some degree of memory impairment. Such impairments are more noticeable with increasing age and severity of the depression. Occasionally the effects upon memory function can be so severe that the person may seem, superficially at least, to be suffering from dementia, which has led to the coining of the term 'pseudodementia'. Other psychiatric disorders such as schizophrenia and anxiety may also cause pseudodementia, but depression is the most common cause.

The classical depressive pseudodementia is caused by a severe major depression, and although the cognitive impairment resolves with treatment of the depression there is a high relapse rate and in many cases it may not fully resolve. Sometimes the residual impairment is age-related and benign, at other times it may be due to coexisting brain disease such as stroke or Parkinson's disease. Furthermore, while in persons under 60 there does not seem to be an increased risk for the later development of dementia, in people older than 60, approximately 25 to 50 per cent develop dementia within three to five years.[3]

The foundation professor of psychiatry at the University of New South Wales in Sydney, Leslie Kiloh, wrote the seminal paper on pseudodementia in 1961. He stressed that in these patients 'the picture of dementia may be very closely mimicked and they may be in danger of therapeutic neglect' and that 'every time the diagnosis of dementia is being considered, the possibility of depression is worth bearing in mind'.[4]

To fully understand the historical context, it needs to be appreciated that in the early 1960s all cases of dementia were considered irreversible. Senile dementia was regarded as either a normal part of ageing or due to arteriosclerosis ('hardening of the arteries'), thus investigation of the cause was not routinely undertaken except in younger people. Consequently, the prospect of older people with undiagnosed depression left lingering untreated in an asylum because they had been mistakenly diagnosed with dementia was not far-fetched. Today this would be an extremely unlikely circumstance, due to the better education of health professionals and the community and the extensive assessment process that is required before people are admitted into residential care.

A more common situation today concerns the person diagnosed with dementia complicated by depression, where it is uncertain how much of the symptoms is due to depression (and hence potentially amenable to antidepressant therapy) and how much is due to dementia. This raises questions about how far trials of treatment should go. Sometimes there is no clear answer to the therapeutic dilemma.

'Reversible' causes of dementia

With the recognition that depression and normal pressure hydrocephalus could present, albeit only occasionally, in a similar fashion to typical cases of senile dementia, researchers around the world began to conduct thorough investigations of patients referred to specialist centres for assessment of dementia or memory impairment. Numerous studies in the 1970s and 1980s reported that up to 17 per cent of people referred for assessment of dementia had potentially reversible conditions. These studies have been very influential on current clinical practice, for the ubiquitous 'dementia screen' of investigations outlined in Table 6.3 was derived from them.

I published a review of these studies in 1991 and concluded that while many medical disorders caused cognitive impairment, most reported cases failed to meet the diagnostic criteria for dementia. Those which did meet the criteria infrequently recovered. Improvements in mental function generally occurred when diagnostic criteria for dementia were not met, the duration of symptoms was less than six months and there was only a mild degree of cognitive impairment. Only 3 per cent of patients diagnosed with dementia fully recovered; of these about two-thirds were either depressed or affected by prescription drugs, usually psychotropic medication. Indeed, in only 5 per cent of all cases assessed as dementia did investigations discover treatable conditions that resulted in cognitive improvement.[5]

Most cases of 'reversible dementia' do not actually have dementia. The correct diagnostic terminology would in many cases be *delirium*, which is a global disorder of cognition that develops over days to weeks and is characterised by fluctuations in alertness, changes in the sleep–wake cycle, poor concentration and memory, visual hallucinations and motor changes of restlessness or apathy. It is when a sub-acute delirium develops over weeks to a few months that a dementia-like state can occur, due, for example to the gradual accumulation of psychotropic drugs such as antidepressants and sedatives.

This does not mean the investigations are unnecessary—they are essential in obtaining an accurate diagnosis; frequently, coincidental medical disorders are discovered that require treatment. Table 6.3 summarises the investigations that are essential and those that are used in select cases. Brain scans allow the clinician to view the brain in three dimensions and see its internal structures. There are many types of brain scans, the most commonly used being the computerised tomography (CT) scan. It takes around 20 minutes to complete and most people with dementia are able to tolerate it. Some clinicians insist on using a magnetic resonance imaging (MRI) brain scan instead, as it provides better quality images, especially if very small lesions, for example, little strokes, are expected. However, in most cases an MRI is not essential. As it involves lying in an enclosed cylinder it can aggravate claustrophobia and some people become quite frightened during the procedure. People with cardiac pacemakers or other metallic implants are unable to be given MRI scans due to the effects of the magnetism on their implants.

Other investigations which have no routine clinical role in the diagnosis of dementia are mainly used in research settings; examples include positron emission tomography (PET) scans and single photon emission computed tomograpy (SPECT) scans, which are used to measure brain function, and genetic screening.

Normal ageing

While it may seem strange to include normality within the differential diagnosis of dementia, this is not too uncommon a finding in older people referred for dementia assessment. About 3 per cent of persons assessed at the Caulfield Cognitive Dementia and Memory Service have been reported to fit this category. The typical 'normal' older person who is referred (usually at their own insistence) for dementia assessment is a rather anxious individual who is well informed about Alzheimer's disease, has become aware of changes in their memory function and fears the worst. When a thorough examination reveals that they are functioning normally, albeit in a manner tainted by anxiety, reassurance that their mental function is normal often suffices. Of course, one can never be absolute in such reassurance, and I usually suggest that they return for a check-up in twelve months, for there is a fine line between normality and mild cognitive impairment.

Mild cognitive impairment

Most people with Alzheimer's disease experience a subtle cognitive decline before reaching the clinical threshold of symptoms that enables diagnosis. Mild cognitive impairment (MCI) refers to this transitional state between normal ageing and mild dementia. This condition has been characterised only in the past decade, so relatively little is known about it and there is still scientific debate about its validity.

Most research to date has focused on those individuals who present with a subjective memory complaint and have an objective memory impairment compared with normal persons of the same age and educational background. While not essential to the diagnosis, it is preferable for the change in memory function to be corroborated by an informant. These individuals are, however, performing reasonably well on indices of general cognitive function and have generally preserved activities of daily living. Persons diagnosed with MCI will need to be reviewed at least annually, undergoing repeat cognitive testing and possibly repeat CT/MRI scans to determine whether there is any progressive brain atrophy, particularly around the hippocampus.[6]

Focal organic brain syndromes

Focal organic brain syndromes occur when only a discrete part of the brain is damaged. They are distinct from dementia because they lack the global disturbances of brain function and are not usually progressive. They can often be severely disabling in their own right, however, and at times the diagnostic distinction will not alter either many aspects of the person's capacity or the type of care required.

Dysmnestic (or *amnestic*) *syndromes* are mainly characterised by profound impairments of short-term memory without other cognitive changes. The most frequently cited cause of dysmnestic syndrome is Wernicke-Korsakoff disorder, which is due to thiamine deficiency damaging the hippocampus, a part of the brain critical for short-term memory function. While alcohol abuse is the most common cause of this disorder, most cases due to alcohol are not 'pure' dysmnestic syndromes insofar as alcohol also damages the frontal lobe of the brain. Often the term 'alcohol-related brain damage' is used to reflect this combination of disorders, thus avoiding the diagnosis of dementia. This type of brain damage has been most commonly recognised as a cause of dementia by Aboriginal people. Other causes of dysmnestic syndromes include pituitary tumours, carbon monoxide poisoning, herpes simplex encephalitis and brain trauma.

Frontal lobe syndromes from damage to the frontal lobe of the brain commonly occur due to excessive alcohol intake (three or more standard drinks per day in a woman, four or more in a man) but are also caused by brain tumours (particularly meningiomas), strokes and subdural haematomas (blood clots) located in this region. Frontal lobe damage is liable to result in behavioural changes, with the precise pattern of symptoms depending on the part of the frontal lobe involved. There are three general patterns: an apathetic, dulled, unmotivated, depressive pattern; a disinhibited, jocular, child-like pattern with poor self-control; and a pattern with poor organisational and planning skills and impaired abstract conceptualisation. Impaired insight and judgement occur to some extent in all three patterns.

Treatment of the cause of the focal brain syndrome usually results in a stable but unremitting impairment. Severely disabled individuals may require long-term residential care, while the moderately impaired usually need some level of ongoing external support from family, friends and community services.

MAKING THE DIAGNOSIS

As the diagnosis of dementia is made on the clinical examination, the examination should be based on well-established diagnostic criteria, either the International Classification of Diseases (ICD-10) or the American Psychiatric Association's *Diagnostic and Statistical Manual* (*DSM-IV*). Once the dementia diagnosis has been made, the type of dementia needs to be determined, and here investigation may identify some concurrent disorder, for example, stroke or thyroid deficiency. Currently there is no available test (blood, urine, CSF, neuro-imaging) that can confirm the diagnosis of Alzheimer's disease in life, though some have been promoted from time to time. In the 1990s, a pupillary dilation test was promoted as being diagnostic for Alzheimer's disease, but this proved to be false. Hence the diagnosis must be based on the presence of typical clinical features and the absence of other identifiable causes. The definitive diagnosis of Alzheimer's disease requires the demonstration of typical neuropathology in brain tissue. As this can only be obtained in life through brain biopsy, confirmation of the diagnosis usually occurs only at autopsy.

The convention is thus to use the term '*probable* Alzheimer's disease' where diagnostic criteria are met and all other possible causes of dementia are eliminated, and '*possible* Alzheimer's disease' where diagnostic criteria are met and another possible cause of dementia is present but judged not to be the main factor, for example, mild vitamin B_{12} deficiency. In centres routinely involved in dementia assessment, these two clinical diagnoses have been found to be about 90 per cent accurate.

In most cases the definitive assessment process may take two or three visits to complete, though this may be lessened if the GP has completed the essential investigations before referral to the specialist. Sometimes symptoms are so mild that a firm diagnosis cannot be made and ongoing review over the following six to twelve months is arranged.

When dementia is confirmed and the type identified through the history, examination and investigations, the next question is:

Should the person with dementia be told the diagnosis? The handling of this issue has changed considerably over time. Twenty years ago, standard practice would have been to tell only the family, unless the dementing person asked to be told what was wrong or had such a mild disorder that it was difficult to avoid telling them. Even in these circumstances, full disclosure of the diagnosis would have been the exception rather than the rule.

Current standard practice is first to ascertain how much the dementing person wants to know about what is wrong. In my experience the majority want to be told the diagnosis, although in some cultures this is not the case. The wish to be told the truth comes about partly because we are seeing more people with milder dementias, and partly because of changed community knowledge and attitudes towards health care. There are a number of good reasons for disclosing the diagnosis. It allows the person with dementia to be involved in planning for their future by preparing wills, arranging an enduring power of attorney and possibly enduring guardianship. It gives them the opportunity to utilise their remaining years of relatively intact cognition in the way that they choose. Of course, it also allows the dementing person to participate actively in treatment planning and, if interested, to participate in dementia support groups. The Alzheimer's Association, which also notes that in more advanced dementia the disclosure of the diagnosis may be neither warranted nor meaningful, supports this general approach.[7]

Giving the diagnosis must be done sensitively, allowing time for the dementing person to assimilate the information. I usually introduce the topic bit by bit, initially by describing the abnormalities found; if the dementing person appears to be becoming distressed, I curtail the extent of information I provide. Often it is the family members who have greatest difficulty with this process, however. Some would rather their relative not be told, for fear of the adverse effect knowing the diagnosis may have. In my experience, adverse reactions are quite uncommon, though occasionally some people become depressed. For some others it may be devastating news that they just cannot tolerate. However, the initial reaction is often one of relief, that there is an explanation for what has been happening to them. Disclosure should be followed up over succeeding visits, however, to ensure that the dementing person is still coping with the bad news.

Eighty-year-old Virginia had been aware that there was something wrong with her memory for some months, though her daughter Penny had been concerned for over a year. The memory clinic had been a daunting experience, and although Virginia couldn't quite remember the precise difficulties she had had with the tests, she knew she had been a little embarrassed about being unable to do them all. Virginia had liked to think that her memory problems were due to her age, but now she was not so sure. When the clinic doctor asked her if she wanted to know what was wrong, she immediately replied, 'Of course.' After some explanation of what the tests had shown, she was told that her memory problems were due to Alzheimer's disease. When asked if she understood what the condition was, she recalled that Ronald Reagan had been diagnosed with it but did not know much else. Penny obviously knew a bit more, for she looked rather wan.

It is often the children of the dementing person who express the most concerns at this point. These include the prospects for treatments that might help, fears about their own prospects of developing a dementia and worries about how their aged parent(s) will cope. The spouse of the dementing person may hold similar concerns, but is often not as vocal. It is critical to provide the family with sufficient information, without overloading them, to allow them to assist in short-term decision making, for example on treatment options. Health department, pharmaceutical company and Alzheimer's Association brochures about aspects of dementia and its treatment should be provided for the family to read in their own time. I usually direct the family to the Alzheimer's Association website where numerous help sheets can be downloaded (see Appendices 1 and 2).

INITIAL MANAGEMENT

It is impossible to separate dementia assessment from initial management, so I will briefly canvass that topic here. Initial medical management should include cognitive enhancing drugs if the diagnosis is Alzheimer's disease and/or dementia with Lewy bodies (see Chapter 5). If there are significant behavioural or psychological complications of the dementia, such as depression, hallucinations or aggression, various psychotropic drugs could be used (see Chapter 7) or psychosocial treatments recommended (see Chapter 8).

Aside from these treatments, the dementing person and their family should be encouraged to plan for the future by making sure that they have a valid will, enduring power of attorney and possibly enduring guardianship in place. If they are still driving, a driving assessment, preferably with an occupational therapist, should be recommended to determine competence to drive (see Chapter 12). Community support services might be required for the more severely affected, particularly if they live alone and need to take medication.

It is also important to recognise that dementia is a chronic disorder that requires long-term commitment of specialist services that are able to interface with general practitioners and community services. Follow-up arrangements to monitor progress are recommended. Family carers and the dementing person often require support after the diagnosis, either from the social worker on the specialist team or the Alzheimer's Association.[8]

SUMMARY

The assessment of dementia ranges from initial detection of cognitive change to the full medical, psychological and social evaluation required to make an accurate diagnosis, address any active psychosocial problems, educate the family and commence appropriate treatments. This process is often enhanced by the involvement of a multidisciplinary team.

CHAPTER 7

DRUG TREATMENTS

TREMENDOUS ADVANCES HAVE TAKEN place over the last five years in the drug treatments of dementia. Yet what has been achieved is merely the tip of the iceberg; much more research will be needed before a cure can be proclaimed for any of the dementing disorders. Current treatments are aimed at ameliorating the symptoms of dementia rather than targeting the underlying causes. Except for a few treatments for specific disorders, current available drug treatments are used across most types of dementia. Here I consider the main domains of treatment and discuss the different options in each domain. As it is not my intent to provide a 'how to' guide for the management of dementia, I give a broad overview of the different drug types rather than providing a great deal of detail on how to use specific drugs. However, I go into some detail on the cholinesterase-inhibitor drugs, due to the stringent Australian Pharmaceutical Benefits Scheme (PBS) regulations.

SOME GENERAL PRINCIPLES

All drugs have side-effects of some sort; in people with dementia increased confusion is common. As the number of drugs prescribed increases, the risk of confusion increases. Drugs that are used in the treatment of dementia may take many weeks to show a positive effect, so providing there are no obvious side-effects, it is important to give each treatment an adequate trial. However, where a drug causes significant side-effects before a positive effect can be determined, it is probably best to discontinue it. In making such a decision the potential, and often intangible, long-term benefits need to be considered, and the decision is not always easy.

MEMORY AND COGNITION: THE COGNITIVE (MEMORY) ENHANCING DRUGS

As memory impairment is the central disturbance of most demen-tias, for many people sustained reversal of the memory disorder is seen as the hallmark of successful treatment. With the knowledge that acetylcholine is critical to memory function and other cogni-tions, and that acetylcholine is deficient in Alzheimer's disease, efforts to rectify the deficit have been the focus of much pharma-ceutical company research over the last 20 years. Attempts to increase the production of acetylcholine in the brain were largely unsuccessful, in part because most drugs were intolerable. It was only when efforts switched to preserving the acetylcholine still present in the brain that progress was made.

Cholinesterase inhibitors

Drugs of the type known as cholinesterase inhibitors have been the only ones to receive approval in Australia for the treatment of mild to moderate Alzheimer's disease. An important issue to note is that these drugs have received approval only for the treatment of Alzheimer's disease, not any other form of dementia, simply because all the major research trials involved only people with Alzheimer's disease when the evidence supporting their use was put to the Food and Drug Administration (FDA) in the United States and Therapeutic Goods Administration (TGA) in Australia. This may change, with research starting to be published on dementia with Lewy bodies and vascular dementia that indi-cates likely benefit from this class of drug.

Cholinesterase inhibitors slow the breakdown of acetylcholine in the nerve synapse, thus increasing the amount available for communication between nerve cells. The first drug to receive marketing approval in the United States and Australia was tacrine (Cognex), which was released in Australia in 1993. Its release was somewhat controversial, as it has very high rates of side-effects, mainly gastrointestinal disturbances and liver toxicity, that limit its use to the extent that relatively few people are able to tolerate a dose sufficient to obtain much benefit. Those able to tolerate it at the highest strength (around one-third of patients) had about 50 per cent chance of obtaining significant improvement of memory function for around a year. Although tacrine is still available in Australia, it is rarely prescribed now that better agents are available.

The second drug released in Australia was donepezil (Aricept) in 1997. It has numerous advantages over tacrine, including relatively low rates of side-effects and once-daily dosing as compared with the four times a day regime of tacrine. Donepezil has subsequently dominated the market in Australia despite the release of two other agents, rivastigmine (Exelon) in 2000 and galantamine (Reminyl) in 2001, both of which have also obtained PBS listing. It should be noted that there is no good evidence that there is any significant difference in the effectiveness of these three drugs.[1]

So, how well do the newer cholinesterase inhibitors work? Put simply, about one-third of Alzheimer patients will have a temporary improvement for approximately twelve to eighteen months, one-third will stabilise for about the same time, and the rest will obtain little if any benefit. There is some emerging evidence that some people may benefit for three or more years, but it is unclear how often this might happen. There are no established predictors as to which people might benefit. An important issue with these drugs is that benefits are maintained only so long as the person keeps taking them. Within a fortnight of cessation, a person who has shown improvement will decline to the presumed level of function that would have occurred without treatment. Thus it is critical that the drugs are taken reliably, as too many missed doses are likely to negate any benefit.

As Table 7.1 shows, gastrointestinal side-effects are the most common side-effects reported, and tend to be the main reason that drugs are not tolerated. Generally speaking, therapeutic doses of donepezil and galantamine are well tolerated; this is not as often the case with rivastigmine.

What do we mean by improvement? Signs of improvement generally emerge within two or three months, though evidence of stabilisation may require at least twelve months of observation. Symptomatic improvement may occur in a number of domains but the most frequently reported areas are better concentration and alertness, improved short-term memory, better global function, improved functional capacity and improved behaviour. This may translate to fewer burdens on family carers. Not all people will benefit in all domains; some people are more alert and show

Table 7.1 Cholinesterase-inhibitor drugs available in Australia

	Tacrine (Cognex)	Donepezil (Aricept)	Rivastigmine (Exelon)	Galantamine (Reminyl)
Effective daily dose range	80–160 mg; much greater response at higher dose	5–10 mg; slightly better response at 10 mg	6–12 mg; ineffective under 6 mg; much greater response at 12 mg	8–24 mg; PBS only supports up to 16 mg, as adverse effects above 16 mg may outweigh benefits
Dosing regime	4 times per day	Once daily (evening)	Twice daily	Twice daily
Severity of side-effects	++++	+	++	+
Types of side-effects	Nausea, vomiting, diarrhoea, fatigue, muscle aches, dizziness, weight loss; liver toxicity is major problem	Nausea, vomiting, diarrhoea, fatigue, dizziness, vivid dreams; occasionally slow heart rate, seizures, bladder neck obstruction; no liver toxicity	Nausea, vomiting, diarrhoea, fatigue, dizziness, headaches; occasionally slow heart rate, seizures, bladder neck obstruction; no liver toxicity	Nausea, vomiting, diarrhoea, fatigue, somnolence, agitation, anorexia; occasionally slow heart rate, seizures, bladder neck obstruction; no liver toxicity
Tolerability	Poorly tolerated, numerous drop-outs	Well tolerated, few drop-outs	Moderately well tolerated, about one-quarter drop-out	Well tolerated up to 16 mg per day

a greater interest in activities but do not appear to have any changes in memory. Others have memory improvements but do not seem to benefit in other ways. How long benefits may last is unpredictable.

This variability in types of treatment responses is of great importance in Australia, where the PBS has placed certain restrictions on the drug subsidies to the public.[2] These are outlined in Table 7.2.

Quite reasonably, the PBS conditions are intended to restrict subsidies to those people who demonstrate response to the drugs. However, that response has been defined almost entirely by improvement in cognitive functioning, with no recognition of any improvements that could occur in global function or behaviour. Just as importantly, as Alzheimer's disease is progressive and on average results in a two or three point reduction on the Mini Mental State Examination (MMSE) every year, clinicians regard lack of decline over a year as a treatment response. Thus, under condition 3, some people who may be benefiting from treatment may lose their PBS subsidy.

While there must be a diagnosis of Alzheimer's disease, it should be noted that if there are good clinical grounds to believe that Alzheimer's disease is co-morbid with another type of dementia, the drugs may be prescribed. As it is highly likely that there is co-morbid Alzheimer's disease in most cases of dementia with Lewy bodies and in cases of vascular dementia where there has been gradual progression, most of these patients thus qualify for a trial.

What can be done to maximise chances of response as defined by the PBS? Most people who respond to cholinesterase inhibitors have either responded after three months or are showing promising signs of response though some may take the full six months allowed. Around 50 to 60 per cent of the patients I treat qualify for the ongoing subsidy. Other clinicians have anecdotally reported similar results. The availability of treatment alternatives and recent changes in the regulations now mean that a second six-month trial can commence after the first six-month trial has failed, and initial non-responders are being given a second and sometimes a third chance.

For how long should these drugs be taken? Basically, cholinesterase inhibitors should be maintained for as long as the

Table 7.2 Australian PBS regulations for the prescription of cholinesterase-inhibitor drugs

1. Diagnosis of mild-moderate Alzheimer's disease
2. Diagnosis confirmed by a specialist (psychiatrist, psychogeriatrician, geriatrician, neurologist, physician)
3. Demonstration of improved cognitive functioning *within six months* of prescription based on standardised cognitive tests performed initially at baseline in either one of these three categories:
    (a) If baseline Mini Mental State Examination (MMSE) score is from 10–24 inclusive, a 2-point improvement is required.
    (b) If baseline MMSE is greater than 24, an ADAS-Cog examination needs to be performed and then a 4-point improvement (which on this scale is a *lower* score) is required.
    (c) If baseline MMSE is less than 10 *and* it is felt that this is partly due to the person having any of the following: poor English language skills; being an Aboriginal/Torres Strait Islander who is unable to do the MMSE for cultural reasons; less than six years' education; illiteracy; innumeracy; disproportionately severe language impairment due to the dementia; severe sensory impairment; or having pre-morbid intellectual impairment; then a Clinician's Interview-Based Impression of Change Scale (CIBIC) can be used and the person needs to be rated at least 'much improved'.
4. Baseline assessments need to be mailed to the PBS before scripts are approved.
5. Six months' supply of cholinesterase-inhibitor drugs is allowed.
6. If there is the defined improvement within the first six months, indefinite PBS subsidy is provided once the PBS receives a letter, accompanying the prescription, that details evidence of the response.
7. Ongoing PBS script approvals (and dose alterations within the first six months) can be by the general practitioner and by phone.
8. Persons who fail to demonstrate the defined improvement within the first six months may embark on a trial of a second cholinesterase inhibitor under the same conditions previously described.

Source: MIMS Australia, Issue No. 1, 2003, p. 103

perceived benefit outweighs any side-effects. There will be an inevitable decline in function for all patients eventually, but this in itself is not a reason to stop medication. If the person is declining rapidly over six months (and other causes for the deterioration are excluded), it may be worth considering a trial of one of the alternatives. This approach is controversial, with dementia experts evenly split on its value. I have had some success with it, so it is my approach. Others suggest a trial discontinuation of therapy. If no worsening is noted after a fortnight, this means the drug has lost its effect; if the person becomes more confused, less functional or more behaviourally disturbed, this provides evidence that the drug is still working and should be immediately recommenced. Another approach is to wait until the person has been placed into a nursing home, when it is advisable to wait for three months after placement and then do the trial discontinuation.

Ginkgo biloba

As described in Chapter 2, the Chinese herb *Ginkgo biloba* is thought to increase blood circulation to the brain and it is prescribed routinely in Europe for memory problems. In Germany ginkgo extracts (240 mg a day) have been approved to treat Alzheimer's disease. Two reviews of the literature published in recent years have concluded there is modest evidence that it may be beneficial for cognition, without appearing to cause many side-effects. It should be noted that ginkgo may cause gastric bleeding, especially when taken with aspirin. The degree of benefit may be comparable to the cholinesterase inhibitors, though the studies have a number of flaws and the most recent well-designed study from the United States was negative. I do not currently recommend the use of ginkgo to my patients as more needs to be known about the dose that is effective. It is, however, a treatment that could be used in all types of dementia.[3]

Vitamin E

There is some modest evidence that vitamin E may slow down the progression of Alzheimer's disease as defined by institutionalisation, functional decline or death. It is unlikely to improve cognition. Although the dose used in the trial that was reported to be effective was 1000 international units twice per day, most clinicians recommend half that amount, as there are concerns that vitamin E can promote bleeding in people with vitamin K deficiency. Though often recommended to be taken in combination with a cognitive enhancing drug, studies have failed to demonstrate additional benefit.[4]

Selegiline

This drug is available in Australia for the treatment of Parkinson's disease. There is modest evidence from a number of studies that it can have beneficial effects on memory, mood and behaviour in Alzheimer's disease, but insufficient evidence to recommend it in routine clinical use.[5]

Memantine (Ebixa)

Memantine has neuroprotective properties and has been approved for use in the treatment of dementia in Germany for over ten years. The European Union's Committee for Proprietary Medicinal Products has also recommended that memantine be approved for treatment of moderately severe to severe Alzheimer's disease in the rest of the European Union. It was released in Australia in August 2003 although it does not yet have PBS listing. Memantine appears to protect the brain's nerve cells against glutamate, a neurotransmitter released in excess amounts by cells damaged by Alzheimer's disease and other neurological disorders. Memantine is very well tolerated and can be combined with cholinesterase inhibitors. It appears to have its greatest effect later in the disease process.[6]

COGNITIVE (MEMORY) ENHANCING DRUGS NOT YET AVAILABLE IN AUSTRALIA

Propentofylline

Propentofylline is regarded as a neuroprotective agent because it inhibits the activation of glial cells, which have a role in causing brain cell destruction. Its use is not tied to any specific type of dementia, and there is evidence of modest efficacy in both Alzheimer's disease and vascular dementia. It could potentially be used in combination with the cholinesterase inhibitors.

Huperzine A

This is a moss extract which has been used in traditional Chinese medicine for centuries. It has properties similar to the established cholinesterase-inhibitor drugs and clinical trials have shown potency similar to these drugs. The main problem is that huperzine A is manufactured without uniform standards, being regarded as a dietary supplement, and this may result in variation in strength from one batch to the next. Huperzine A should not be used in combination with approved cholinesterase inhibitors as there is potential for adverse drug–drug interactions.[7]

SOME UNPROVEN COGNITIVE (MEMORY) ENHANCING DRUGS

Brahmi

This is an Ayurvedic herb popular in India and Japan as a nerve tonic for treating insomnia and nervous tension, and for improving memory. There is no good evidence that it is of any benefit in the treatment or prevention of dementia.

GH3 (Gerovital)

This procaine-based agent, also known as KH3, is heavily promoted as an 'anti-ageing nutrient' which, amongst many claims, may assist 'failing memory' and 'senility'. There is no good evidence that it is of any benefit in the treatment or prevention of dementia, though some people report that they feel less depressed.

Phosphatidylserine

This is a type of fat found in cell membranes and is supposed to protect cells from damage by bolstering the cell membrane. As this substance was derived from the brain cells of cows, the outbreak of 'mad cow disease' effectively ended investigations, although early clinical trials showed some interesting results.

Drugs for the behavioural and psychological symptoms of dementia

Behavioural changes such as agitation, aggression, sexual disinhibition and disruptive vocalisations, alongside psychological symptoms such as depression, anxiety, paranoid delusions and hallucinations, are often the most distressing part of the dementing process for both carers and the person with dementia. The International Psychogeriatric Association has coined the umbrella term 'behavioural and psychological symptoms of dementia' (BPSD) to describe these clinical features. Other terms that have been used include 'problem behaviours', 'disruptive behaviours' and 'challenging behaviours', the last of these being preferable as it suggests that most behaviours involve an interaction between the carer and the dementing person. I prefer the term 'BPSD', as it includes the psychological component. BPSD has been found to be the major factor contributing to stress in family and professional carers and to the dementing person being placed into institutional care. In essence, the carer gets burnt out from dealing with BPSD.[8]

Many different psychotropic drugs (drugs used to treat psychiatric disorders) have been used with varying degrees of success to treat the problems of BPSD. In fact, one of the major issues that has arisen worldwide, particularly in nursing homes, is the overuse and misuse of these drugs. In research that I undertook with Henry Brodaty in 1996–97 in eleven Sydney nursing homes, we found that 59 per cent of residents (most of whom had dementia) had been prescribed at least one psychotropic drug in the previous month, and 22 per cent had been prescribed two or more. About 30 per cent were prescribed sleeping tablets, 25 per cent antipsychotic drugs and 20 per cent antidepressants. Importantly, we found that those prescribed antidepressants had the highest rates of depression and those prescribed antipsychotics the highest rates of psychosis. It appeared that the correct types of drugs were being prescribed but that their effectiveness was questionable.[9]

This raises the fundamental issue in the management of BPSD. It is important to realise that just because a dementing person has a certain behaviour or psychological symptom, this does not automatically mean that it should be treated. Unless BPSD is distressing the dementing person or causing significant problems for others around them, the situation may be best left as it is. If treatment is required, non-drug (psychosocial) treatments should always be considered first; even if drugs are used, non-drug treatments will usually be needed in combination. All such drugs should be prescribed at the lowest effective dose. I consider psychosocial treatments in Chapter 8.

Another important issue is consent for treatment. (I consider the broader issue of mental competence and the determination of capacity in Chapter 12.) As the majority of dementing people prescribed psychotropics for BPSD will have lost their capacity to consent, it is essential that legal consent be obtained. The precise process varies from state to state in Australia and elsewhere. In New South Wales, psychotropic drugs are classified as a 'major medical treatment' and as such require *written consent* from the legally defined 'person responsible'—usually the spouse, child, sibling or legal guardian of the person. It is doubtful that this happens too often, though I suspect verbal consent is obtained in most cases.

A third issue is the use of drugs as a form of chemical restraint—in other words, where psychotropic drugs are used simply to sedate the dementing person rather than being used for their therapeutic effects. Usually this involves excessive dosing, with the dementing person left in an oversedated, drowsy state for most of the time. While this might occur inadvertently during efforts to control severe agitation and aggression, it should only be a transient phase as the correct dose of medication is sought. Chronic oversedation is dangerous, inappropriate, unnecessary and unethical.

Here I will consider some of the more commonly prescribed psychotropic drugs along with the main indications for their use (summarised in Table 7.3).

Antipsychotic drugs

Antipsychotics are primarily designed to treat psychoses such as schizophrenia. For many years they have also been used in the management of dementia, though only in the past five years have a few good studies been completed to determine their effectiveness. As one might expect, psychotic symptoms such as

Table 7.3 Drugs for the behavioural and psychological symptoms of dementia

Type	Examples
Atypical antipsychotics	risperidone (Risperdal), olanzapine (Zyprexa), quetiapine (Seroquel)
Other ('traditional') antipsychotics	haloperidol (Serenace), trifluoperazine (Stelazine, Calmazine), thioridazine (Aldazine), chlorpromazine (Largactil)
SSRI antidepressants	sertraline (Zoloft), citalopram (Cipramil), paroxetine (Aropax, Paxtine, Roxatine), fluoxetine (Prozac, Fluohexal, Zactin, Lovan), fluvoxamine (Luvox)
Other antidepressants	venlafaxine (Efexor), mirtazepine (Avanza, Remeron), moclobemide (Aurorix, Arima, Mohexal, Clobemix)
Mood stabilisers	carbamazepine (Tegretol, Teril), sodium valproate (Epilim, Valpro)
Benzodiazepines	diazepam (Antenex, Ducene, Valium, Valpam), oxazepam (Murelax, Serepax), temazepam (Temaze, Euhypnos, Normison, Nocturne, Temtabs), nitrazepam (Alodorm, Mogadon)
Other sedatives	zopiclone (Imovane), chlormethiazole (Hemineurin)
Hormonal treatments	cyproterone acetate (Androcur, Cyprone, Cyprostat, Climen)

suspiciousness, false beliefs (delusions), accusations, paranoia and hallucinations are the main target. They are also effective in treating aggressive behaviours, agitation and sexual disinhibition. Sometimes they can help disruptive vocalisations.

There are, broadly, two main groups of antipsychotic drugs. The first is the older 'traditional' drugs, of which haloperidol (usual dose range 0.5–3 mg) has the best evidence for effectiveness and is the most widely prescribed. The problem with these drugs is their high rates of side-effects. With haloperidol, for example, around 20 per cent of recipients develop symptoms of parkinsonism at normal therapeutic doses—shuffling gait, stooped posture, slowed movements and increased risk of falls. Other problems include increased confusion, oversedation and constipation. After a few months use, all drugs in this group have a high risk of causing tardive dyskinesia (abnormal movements with delayed onset), which involves involuntary movements, in particular with the mouth and tongue. It is quite distressing, unsightly and often permanent.

The second group is the 'atypical' antipsychotics. The general advantage of the atypical antipsychotics is their lower rate of side-effects. For example, the parkinsonian side-effects occur in only 2 to 5 per cent of patients and tardive dyskinesia is much less frequent, though the risk of stroke might be increased. Risperidone has the best evidence of effectiveness in dementia, with the world's largest study coordinated in Australia by Henry Brodaty from the University of New South Wales, Sydney. Risperidone is the only drug in this group that has TGA approval for the treatment of dementia in Australia. The usual dose range is 0.5–2 mg per day.

Antipsychotic drugs are best avoided in dementia with Lewy bodies (DLB) due to their propensity to cause severe parkinson-ism in this condition at very low dosage, even the atypical drugs. As hallucinations are common in DLB, treatment is often required; fortunately, the cholinesterase-inhibitor drugs seem to be effective in settling such psychotic symptoms.

The main options from each group, haloperidol and risperi-done, have been compared head to head in a large study and found to have similar effectiveness, with haloperidol having the expected higher rate of side-effects. A major dilemma confronting con-sumers in Australia is that none of the atypical antipsychotic drugs attract a PBS subsidy for the treatment of dementia, but the older drugs do. The atypicals are expensive, with the unsubsidised cost being $60 to $100 per month. The only condition for which the PBS subsidy applies is schizophrenia, and there have been doctors prepared to state to the PBS authorities that their dementing patient has schizophrenia in order for the patient to obtain the subsidy. Doctors caught making false statements to the PBS are liable to heavy penalties. A few years ago a doctor in Queensland was asked to repay over $1 million dollars for making false state-ments to the PBS (about a different type of drug).

My approach is to explain the treatment options to carers along the lines that both types of drug have similar effectiveness, that the cheaper drugs have a higher risk of side-effects, the more expensive drugs a lower risk. By framing the choices in terms similar to other commodities (the principle of you pay for what you get), carers are able to decide what they believe is the best 'value for money'. It should be noted, however, that the majority of patients prescribed the older drugs will *not* get serious side-effects, and that some who are prescribed the newer drugs will. It is a matter of relative risk.

> Roger had always had a short temper but now he seemed to strike out at the least provocation. He seemed suspicious of others and had made no close friends in the nursing home. The nursing staff treated him gingerly as he had clobbered them a few times. Eventually, after numerous efforts to manage him without drugs, a trial of risperidone was commenced. After some weeks Roger was obviously less suspicious and less irritable. His aggressive outbursts were now containable through diversional strategies.

How long should these drugs be prescribed? If the target behaviours or symptoms have remained under control for six months, I recommend a trial discontinuation.

Antidepressant drugs

Antidepressant drugs are mainly used to treat depression and anxiety, but can also be used for disruptive vocalisations, agitation and sleep disturbances. Their effectiveness in treating depression and anxiety associated with dementia is limited, though some good results are obtained. One reason for this is that depression associated with dementia does not always have typical features, so that accurate diagnosis is harder. Another is that the brain damage caused by the dementia inhibits the action of the drugs.

There are many different classes of antidepressants but in general they can be divided into the older drugs, such as the tricyclic antidepressants, and the newer drugs, particularly the selective serotonin reuptake inhibitors (SSRIs). As with the antipsychotic drugs, the main difference between the older and newer drugs is the higher rate of side-effects with the older drugs; there is little difference in the effectiveness of the two groups. Possibly the older drugs work better with very severe depression, but this is rarely an issue in the treatment of dementia.

Experts consistently recommend the SSRI antidepressants as the first line of treatment of depression and anxiety in older people, whether or not these conditions are associated with dementia. The drugs of choice are usually sertraline (25–100 mg per day) and cipramil (10–30 mg per day), which have been shown to be effective in depression associated with dementia and have the lowest risk of drug interactions. All SSRIs can have side-effects that include nausea, vomiting, diarrhoea, agitation and falls. There is also a risk of sodium depletion, which may cause confusion, lethargy and weakness, so the person's sodium levels need to be checked. One concern expressed in some quarters about sertraline is the possibility that it might unleash sudden irrational behaviour, as evidenced by one older man who committed murder after taking a higher than prescribed dose in combination with alcohol. I doubt whether any specific property of sertraline was responsible for this tragedy. If SSRIs are ineffective, the main treatment options are probably venlafaxine, moclobemide or mirtazepine. Antidepressants should generally be prescribed for a minimum of six months if they are effective.[10]

Mood stabilising drugs

These drugs are used to treat epilepsy, chronic pain and bipolar (manic-depressive) illness. The main indications for their use in dementia are aggression, agitation and mood instability. The evidence for their effectiveness is limited to a few studies, but many practitioners find sodium valproate to be very useful with aggressive behaviour. Side-effects are largely related to sedation and unsteady gait, but tend to be dose-related. Serum levels are available to assist in finding the optimal dose.

Sedative-hypnotic and anxiolytic drugs

Most of these drugs are in the benzodiazepine class and are of very limited use in dementia, as they tend to oversedate. There is also the possibility of a paradoxical reaction in which agitation worsens instead of abating. For this reason night sedation is the main indication, and here the short-acting temazepam is the first choice as it is less likely to cause a hangover effect in the morning. Another short-acting non-benzodiazepine that can be useful here is zopiclone (Imovane). Chlormethiazole (Hemineurin) is also used for agitation but is expensive.

Antiandrogens (hormonal treatments)

These are used in men with recalcitrant sexually inappropriate behaviour and/or aggression. The main drug is cyproterone acetate, which works by suppressing testosterone levels. This is a controversial treatment and regarded as second or third line after other treatment trials have failed. In New South Wales, the Guardianship Tribunal has to provide consent for this treatment for a mentally incompetent person, even when there is a legal guardian in place. I have prescribed it several times with success.

Analgesics

I mention analgesics (painkillers) here because pain is a common factor in BPSD and is notoriously poorly treated in older people. Analgesics can range from simple treatments such as aspirin and paracetamol through to narcotic analgesics such as morphine and pethidine. In advanced dementia where communication is limited, a restless bedfast person may well be in serious discomfort but unable to communicate it verbally other than by screaming. Presuming factors such as chronic constipation and other obvious causes of pain have been excluded, a palliative care approach to treatment by using optimal doses of narcotic analgesics to relieve distress without oversedation is sensible.

> Mary had been in the nursing home for eighteen months with advanced dementia. She no longer spoke intelligibly and was bedfast. To the consternation of staff, residents and neighbours, Mary would scream in a loud high-pitched voice for many hours every day. No particular reason could be identified for the noise. She called out whether or not family were present, at all times of the day and night, before and after meals, before and after personal care from nurses. Distraction, attention, touch, aromatherapy and music therapy made no difference. Various antipsychotic and antidepressant drugs had no impact. Simple analgesics were ineffective. Eventually, in desperation, mist morphine was

commenced and within days the noise improved, although it never stopped. The reduction was sufficient for staff and residents to obtain some respite.

MEDICAL PROBLEMS THAT IMPACT ON DEMENTIA

In earlier chapters, I indicated that a range of medical conditions, including hypertension, diabetes mellitus, cardiac disorders, high cholesterol, hypothyroidism and vitamin B_{12} and folate deficiency, may contribute to cognitive changes. It is important that such conditions be optimally treated to maximise function. This will be particularly important in people with vascular dementia. Drugs commonly required include antihypertensives, antiplatelet drugs (aspirin), diuretics and the replacement of all vitamin and hormone deficiencies.

Epileptic fits may occur later in the course of dementia, where anticonvulsant drugs may be needed. Here sodium valproate or carbamazepine may be the drugs of choice due to their potential benefits on behaviour. Urinary incontinence is often a problem that can make or break community care; if this is the case a trial of low dose oxybutynin (Ditropan) might be considered. As it tends to have the opposite effect to the cholinesterase inhibitors it can increase confusion, and so is a treatment to be used cautiously.

SUMMARY

The drug treatment of dementia symptoms has improved considerably in the past decade but as most current treatments have significant shortcomings there is still much room for improvement. There are two main areas of treatment—drugs which target cognition and also seem to benefit behaviour and function, and drugs which target the behavioural and psychological symptoms of dementia.

CHAPTER 8

PSYCHOSOCIAL TREATMENTS

DEMENTIA CAN BE SUCH a distressing condition that the importance of continuing to 'live life' is lost to many people. This is a complex topic that has many nuances.

Whole books have been written about how to interact with persons with dementia. In this chapter, rather than writing a condensed version of one of the excellent books that have a practical 'how to' focus (see list in Appendix 3), I outline common psychosocial approaches that are utilised in dementia care, most of which are based upon the achievement of well-being. The themes that emerge will hopefully provide some guidance about living with dementia.

SOME GENERAL RULES OF COMMUNICATION

There are some general rules about communication with a person with dementia that are worth mentioning. Remember that the person is dement*ing*, not dement*ed*. This means that many mental functions remain relatively intact until the later stages of illness, and these retained abilities should be tapped into *as much as possible.* Another common mistake that carers and other people make is to talk down to the person as if they were a child or not present at all. Such an approach is both demeaning and likely to provoke resentment. Try to communicate on an adult–adult level but keep things simple. Short sentences containing only one subject are better than longer ones. When asking questions, avoid the 'multiple choice' approach. For example, rather than asking 'Would you like to go to the movies, go to the concert or out to a restaurant?', it would be better to break down the question into two or three parts. Use gestures, speak slowly and clearly but try not to be stilted.

EARLY DEMENTIA

I am not exactly sure how I would react if I was told I had Alzheimer's disease. Maybe I would be like many of my better informed patients these days, who already suspect the diagnosis and to whom its confirmation comes as no surprise. That doesn't mean that the diagnosis isn't upsetting, but at least it removes uncertainty and provides an opportunity to plan for the future. There are many other types of reactions. It might be depressing, as any bad news would be, but most people want to face it and not avoid it. To some, however, it may be absolutely devastating. Some people acknowledge the diagnosis, then simply forget what they have been told, or go into denial about it. Others just don't want to know, but that reaction is uncommon.

Emotional support and lifestyle advice

Most people want their family, close friends and doctor to be emotionally supportive during this period. Support groups for persons with early dementia are becoming increasingly common as more people in our ageing population are being diagnosed earlier in the course of their illness. Tom Kitwood, who has written extensively on this topic, uses the term 'holding' as a metaphor for providing a safe place where frightening emotions can be experienced without the dementing person being overwhelmed by them.[1]

For health care professionals, the technical terms used for emotional support are 'supportive psychotherapy' and 'counselling'. These psychological therapies are simply intended to allow the recipient an opportunity to ventilate their feelings with an attentive, empathic person who is non-judgemental in the support they provide. Some basic advice and information about planning for the future and for legal decisions, as described in Chapter 6, may be given as part of the process of assisting the dementing person in adjusting to their changed circumstances.

One piece of advice that I regularly offer is encouraging the dementing person and their family to maintain as much of their usual lifestyle for as long as possible. Tom Kitwood uses the term 'celebration' to describe the various simple activities that the dementing person can enjoy with friends and family to maintain life—singing, walking, eating good meals. Some precautions may need to be taken; for example, trips to distant locations may lead to increased confusion so the dementing person should always travel with an informed carer. Yet on the whole, few changes in lifestyle are required for most people with early dementia.

Memory training

People with mild cognitive impairment and mild dementia may benefit from memory training to enhance their residual memory function.[2] Probably the most common strategies taught involve the use of 'external memory aids'. Most of us use external memory aids regularly, for example, diaries, shopping lists, alarm clocks and message boards in the kitchen. For the person with memory deficits who is not in the habit of using any of these aids, the most difficult thing to achieve is the regular use of the aid. This often requires regular input from a carer, as well as from the therapist, to get things going. Using diaries and message boards are probably the most common techniques. Both allow the dementing person and their carers to add items as they arise. Thus a carer might write in the diary the time they are going to pick up the dementing person for a shopping trip, or leave a prominent message on the message board about a forthcoming event. The dementing person is encouraged to write all day-to-day tasks into their diary, including what people tell them on telephone calls. By habitually referring to their memory aids, they can minimise the impact of short-term memory impairment. Another form of external memory aid is the regular phone call from a carer to remind the dementing person to take their tablets, or of an upcoming appointment. This is usually the approach in mild-moderate dementia.

New learning can also be enhanced by the appropriate use of cues. Cues are commonly used in study techniques to improve recall for examinations. Students might use lists, acronyms, pictures, visual imagery and so on when they study. A similar approach can be encouraged to counter mild memory deficits due to dementia. As with study techniques, self-generated cues are more likely to work. The dementing person is asked to think of questions or images to remind them of what they are learning. Such associations assist later recall of the information. Because it is essential not to overload the dementing person with trivial information, this approach is best reserved for the items most important to them. It also needs to be done in a manner that is relaxing and not onerous. When efforts to enhance learning resemble being in school, they are bound to fail, especially if the process becomes anxiety provoking.

Another way of enhancing new learning of specific events is to ensure that the event stands out from the daily routine. Having a daily routine for a dementing person reduces the information load they have to assimilate, and reduces their stress levels. For an important event such as a birthday party, enrichment of the occasion with the dementing person's favourite music, colourful decorations, favourite food and close friends will assist them in remembering the occasion.

Making memories

An interesting project currently being sponsored by the Alzheimer's Association involves persons with early dementia putting together an autobiography that can assist them as the disease progresses. This might involve audiotapes, videotapes, diaries, photos and other bits of nostalgia from their life. As this initiative is quite recent, it is as yet unclear whether it is beneficial or not. Some people might find it a lot of fun, so for those who are interested it seems to me a good idea.

MODERATE–SEVERE DEMENTIA

Numerous therapies have been designed to assist in the communication, stimulation and comforting of people with moderate–severe dementia. Some of the therapies overlap and to date there is not much evidence that any particular approach is more effective than any other. It is most likely that there is a lot of common ground and in part all are likely to work by providing professional and family carers with tools to help them in their interactions with dementing people. The importance of such assistance should not be underestimated, for coping with a dementing person can be an overwhelming prospect for the inexperienced. Choice is probably helpful in itself; being able to tap into a variety of different approaches and therapies may be useful.

Routines are an important feature of most therapies—setting aside a period of time each day to do something can assist in structuring the day for both the dementing person and carer alike. Another thing that must be remembered is that most therapies only have an effect in and around the period of their application. Thus a behavioural disturbance might be settled for the duration of the therapy and an hour or two after, but not much longer. It might be necessary to have another therapy session routinely organised afterwards, possibly of a different type of therapy, to help quell the re-emerging behaviour.

Validation therapy

Naomi Feil developed validation therapy between 1963 and 1980 to assist in communicating with people who have dementia and other disorders with cognitive impairment.[3] It is a humane, practical approach that emphasises stage-specific communication techniques. The principal assumption underlying validation therapy is that all behaviour has meaning, even if the behaviour is extremely inappropriate or based on psychotic experiences. Its main technique is to validate the dementing person's emotions by acknowledging their feelings, even when they may be based on misinterpretations or misperceptions. The goal of therapy is to make the dementing person as happy as possible.

Meg was experiencing hallucinations in which she saw masked intruders come into her room. She worried that they might assault her and thus screamed in distress. The first nurse who responded tried to reassure her by telling her that she was just imagining the men and so she wouldn't be at any risk. Meg remained very scared and kept screaming. A second nurse comforted her by saying 'It must be very scary to have strange men in your room', which allowed Meg to agree and describe how terrified she had been. Eventually Meg calmed down and seemed more at ease.

The second nurse used a validation therapy approach to communication. By acknowledging Meg's fear, this nurse demonstrated empathy with Meg's plight. The type of reassurance offered by the first nurse had the unintended effect of invalidating Meg's emotions. In reasonably insightful people who experience hallucinations, reassurance that the hallucinations are not real *might* work, providing that acknowledgement of how distressing the hallucinations are accompanies the reassurance.

Feil classifies individuals with cognitive impairment as being at one of four stages on a continuum of dementia. These stages are 'malorientation', 'time confusion', 'repetitive motion' and 'vegetation', all occurring in the moderate and severe stages of dementia. While validation therapy was not designed for mild dementia, the basic technique of validating the person's emotions is derived from counselling psychology and would still be applicable. In general, validation therapy aims to work with the dementing person's spared abilities and functions while bolstering those that are more severely affected.

Feil describes numerous benefits of validation therapy. These include restoration of the self-worth of the dementing person, minimisation of the degree to which dementing people withdraw from the outside world, promotion of communication and interaction with other people, reduction of stress and anxiety, stimulation of dormant potential, help in resolving unfinished life tasks and facilitation of independent living for as long as possible. To date, there has been relatively little empirical research to investigate these claims and so the extent to which validation therapy achieves these benefits is unknown. A major problem is that research in this area is very difficult to undertake in a fashion that would satisfy most academics that the therapy has a specific benefit (as opposed to the non-specific benefit of having carers providing a similar level of any interaction with the dementing person). However, descriptive research that has observed validation therapy being used, and anecdotal experience, suggest that there are positive effects.

There are a number of criticisms of validation therapy.[4] Possibly the most common is that some carers find this style of communication very difficult to use, because they feel that they are 'colluding' with delusions. Carers who must be 'right' or be 'in control' seem to have the most problems, particularly where the relationship with the dementing person was marked by confrontation before the onset of dementia. Others say that validation therapy is more an attitude towards caregiving than a formal therapy. To me, the general approach appears very sensible, non-confrontational and positive.

Reminiscence therapy

Robert Butler first described reminiscence or 'life review' therapy in 1963. It is based on the premise that reminiscence is beneficial for people in the later stages of their life because it provides them with an opportunity to review and reorganise the events of their life in response to the biological and psychological fact of impending death. From this it can be seen that reminiscence therapy is not specifically designed for persons with dementia; indeed, it has been used more frequently to treat depression, to assist in socialisation and as an aid for successful ageing.[5]

In people with dementia, the goals of reminiscence therapy are to decrease isolation and improve morale and well-being by triggering memories of previous life events. It is usually conducted in a group setting on a weekly basis, often in a day care centre, hostel or nursing home. Music and other cues such as photos, videos and books are used to trigger memories. The choice of cues should be relevant to group members, thus the group leader will require information on the group members' backgrounds. There is evidence that reminiscence therapy can reduce depressive symptoms, improve life satisfaction and facilitate communication. Note, however, that some people may not be suited to reminiscence therapy, particularly those who have endured horrific life experiences such as the Holocaust.

It is a technique that can be used in interactions with moderate to severely impaired dementing people, as a way of stimulating pleasant memories, possibly as a distraction when the dementing person is upset, or as a way of providing mental stimulation. Some people with mild dementia may use reminiscence techniques as part of a memory training program, for example, in attempting to remember the names of classmates at school.

> Percy had been feeling miserable all day and was quite grumpy whenever his wife Norma tried to find out what was wrong. Eventually she decided to play their favourite song, 'The Girl from Ipanema', and started talking with Percy about the fun times they used to have at Saturday night dances.

Percy seemed to brighten with the music and with a little encouragement started dancing with Norma while reminiscing happily about their courtship.

Reality orientation

Reality orientation was first described in 1966 as a technique to improve the quality of life of confused older people. It is mainly designed for people with moderate–severe dementia and involves the presentation of orientation and memory information in a group or individual setting in order to provide the dementing person with a greater understanding of their surroundings and to improve their sense of control and self-esteem. There are two types of reality orientation therapy—continuous and classroom. Continuous 24-hour reality orientation is mainly practised in residential care settings where staff involve the dementing residents in reality-based communication in every contact throughout the day. Classroom reality orientation is where groups meet on a regular basis to engage in orientation-related activities.[6]

Devices that can be used to assist in the therapy include calendars, clocks, scrapbooks, television and video, educational sessions and newspapers. Typically, there is a noticeboard that displays information, including the weather, day, date and place, forthcoming meals and outings. (Unfortunately, in my experience many noticeboards are not updated with current information, thus defeating their purpose.) All these devices are used to stimulate conversation about what is happening in the 'real' world and to assist in practising skills such as grooming, feeding and socialising. It is a reasonably simple technique that can be adapted to many settings.

Critics of reality orientation claim that it is often applied in a mechanistic fashion that is insensitive to the individual needs of the dementing persons, and that the constant relearning of material may contribute to the lowering of self-esteem and mood. In fact, it was such concerns that contributed to Naomi Feil's development of validation therapy and the loss of popularity of the reality orientation technique. However, there is quite good research evidence that the technique can have beneficial effects on memory, orientation and behaviour, and it may be premature to abandon it. What might be more important is to avoid the rigid application of the therapy without consideration of individual needs.

Music therapy

Music therapy is more than simply playing music in the back-ground for its calming effects. It is a well-established therapy used in the treatment of a range of mental disorders. Music can evoke emotions that may not be easily tapped into through other means. Most of us have experienced the powerful nostalgic reminiscence cued by songs associated with particular events in our life—a tune our parents enjoyed, or the one we first danced to with our spouse are common examples. In people who may be having some diffi-culties in dealing with psychological trauma, music may assist the therapist in helping them talk about it.

For people with dementia, music therapy has two main func-tions. Firstly, it provides a pleasurable experience, through both listening and participation. Regular groups in which the music therapist may play a combination of recorded and live music that allows the participants to listen, sing and play instruments are a feature of many day care centres and aged care facilities. This type of therapy is largely intended to improve quality of life through social interaction and diversion.

The second function is as a specific therapy designed to reduce behavioural disturbances in aged care facilities. Quiet music played during mealtimes can reduce agitation and result in greater compliance with eating. Research has shown that when the indi-vidual's musical preferences are used in a music therapy program (as opposed to no music or a standard musical selection), behav-ioural disturbances are reduced.[7] This may seem self-evident but too often the music played in facilities does not reflect the choices of the residents. Recently I visited a nursing home to advise on the management of a noisy resident. While I was in her room, the radio was booming with rap music that was clearly being enjoyed by the young cleaner but by none of the older residents. (If I had to listen to rap music all day I think I might get quite noisy!)

Physical exercise and activity programs

In Chapter 2, I discussed the potential role of physical exercise in the prevention of dementia. It should come as no surprise that exercise can also be beneficial for dementia sufferers. For the person who has been very physically active through their life, it is important to maintain that activity. Often participation in sports such as golf and lawn bowls wanes as the dementia progresses due to declining skills, loss of initiative and family concerns about safety. Dancing and walking are recreational pursuits that can be maintained for much longer if there is a regular partner who can guide the dementing person. I always encourage participation in a favoured physical activity for as long as possible, even if it requires modification of the dementing person's involvement. Older persons who withdraw from physical activity due to their health often become unhappy and demoralised, and some become clinically depressed.

Physical exercise is also very useful for people who have not been very active over the years and for those who are in nursing homes. The type of activity may need to be varied to suit the individual; if the person has limited mobility, for example, gentle bending and stretching exercises while seated can be beneficial. Whatever type of exercise the dementing person is encouraged to do, the most important thing is that it is enjoyable. Group games with a ball, musical games, dances, walks, aerobics, anaerobics—the list is almost endless. The exercise should also be undertaken regularly, at least 30 minutes per day five times per week. There is good evidence that optimal physical activity can improve sleep patterns, reduce depressive symptoms and settle behavioural disturbances such as agitation, noisiness and aggression.[8]

Non-exercise based activity programs are also important. Singing, art, bingo, television, discussion groups, relaxation therapy and various group games provide mental stimulation to help alleviate boredom and encourage appropriate social interaction in day care centres and aged care facilities. There is overlap between therapies, thus discussion groups may involve reminiscence and reality orientation techniques, and so on.

Aromatherapy and touch therapy

Most people enjoy a pleasant fragrance and a soothing touch. It is little wonder that aromatherapy and touch therapy, including massage, may have a role in dementia care. Both therapies are forms of complementary medicine and have an extensive history and rationale for their use in various conditions. I don't pretend to understand these therapies at that level; I do regard them as having the potential to improve the dementing person's quality of life through the provision of pleasant experiences.

Aromatherapy with essential oils has been used mainly as a calming or relaxing influence during the day and as a mild sedative at night. Essential oils are usually applied by room fragrancers, but they can also be delivered in baths, by massage and through inhalations. Lavender oil is possibly the most frequently used, particularly for sleep disturbances. Sometimes a lavender bag is placed under the pillow. Other commonly used oils include chamomile, bergamot, sandalwood and rose. There is some evidence that aromatherapy works in these situations so it should be considered as a component of the package of care.

We often forget how important it is to have direct human contact. Cuddling and holding hands are more than just displays of affection between lovers. There is evidence that such contact increases brain serotonin levels and helps to make us feel happy and content. Similarly, therapeutic massage not only has a direct effect on the muscles being massaged, it also has a general soothing influence on the mind. Many older people in nursing homes have very little opportunity for such contact and often crave human touch from visitors. Not surprisingly, studies have shown that both hand massage and therapeutic touch reduce agitated behaviours in nursing home residents. Of course, touch and massage don't need to be as formalised as this but simply incorporated within routine care programs as a regular part of day-to-day interaction, providing it is acceptable to the dementing person. A few people prefer not to be touched.[9]

Audiotapes and videotapes

It is a frequent observation in nursing homes that persons with severe dementia are more content when family members are present. Simulated Presence Therapy uses audiotapes prepared by family members about past experiences and other personal nostalgia. The families are instructed to talk to the dementing person on tape and ask questions, leaving gaps so that the dementing person can answer. Although there is currently only limited evidence, it does appear to be an effective therapy for calming agitated behaviours. Often the dementing person is observed to respond to the tape as if the family member were present. The same tape can be used repeatedly, as at the severe stage of dementia it is quickly forgotten. This therapy has many attractions for me. It is sensible, inexpensive and involves the family at a time when many members feel they are unable to contribute much. While I have not seen any reports of using family videos in the same way, this is likely to be another possible application.[10]

I have regularly advised on the use of selected videotapes based upon the dementing person's known interests. Anecdotally, I have observed that videos of favourite sporting events, concerts and, of course, old films can be shown repeatedly and have a calming effect if the choice is right for the individual. If the video is not suited to the individual it is usually of little benefit.

Behaviour therapy

Behaviour therapy is based on learning theory and is used to eliminate unwanted behaviours and to encourage desirable behaviours in people with moderate–severe dementia. There has been much debate about how much can be learnt at this stage of dementia and critics of the therapy claim that it is a fundamentally flawed approach. However, several small Australian studies have demonstrated that sufficient learning can occur to allow for the successful treatment of noisy and intrusive behaviours.[11]

The fundamentals of behaviour therapy are familiar to all of us—rewarding desirable behaviours encourages behaviour change. Most parents use variations of this theme in raising their children. The trick is to work out an appropriate reward for the dementing person that will be sufficient to encourage change. Food, drink and pleasurable activities are the rewards most frequently used, but it may take a while to identify the right reward for the individual.

At the same time, unwanted behaviours should be ignored. The mistake that many people make here is to punish rather than ignore. Punishment should definitely not be a part of a behaviour therapy program. It may be hard to ignore some types of behaviour and it may be difficult for carers to tolerate such behaviours, especially as a behaviour therapy program needs to be applied consistently for some weeks to be effective. Time is often a major limiting factor in the application of behaviour therapy in residential care, as we found in one study of the treatment of noisy nursing home residents in Sydney and Newcastle. Nursing staff reported that behaviour programs were often too time consuming to apply when they were already extremely busy.[12]

Pet therapy

Companion animals have been described as potentially fulfilling a number of functions for older dementing people. They can be objects of affection, empathy and communication, as well as a focal point for group communications and activities in residential care. Benefits may extend to staff, carers and volunteers as well. Socialisation may be improved. Pets do not suit everybody so it is important to identify those who have an aversion to a particular animal. As we all know, there are 'cat people' and 'dog people'. There are also potential dangers, with the possibility of tripping over the animal being a major concern, and the need to supervise well-meaning efforts to care for an animal that may inadvertently harm it. We recently introduced a galah into our ward and within days one woman had been pecked on the finger as she tried to play with it. Fortunately the cut was minor.[13]

Light therapy

It has been postulated that the commonly observed worsening of agitated behaviour in the late afternoon and early evening ('sundowning') may be partially due to changes in circadian sleep–wake cycles. The application of bright fluorescent lights for several hours during the day in an effort to influence these circadian rhythms has been found to have a modest effect on sundowning behaviours in nursing home settings. At this stage, there is insufficient evidence for light therapy to be used as a mainstream treatment, but it might be worth a try with a person whose nocturnal sleep pattern has failed to improve with other treatments.[14]

Multisensory stimulation: Snoezelen rooms

Multisensory stimulation has become very popular in the United Kingdom as a treatment for calming agitation, stimulating those who are withdrawn and encouraging communication with carers. It was initially used for people with learning disabilities but over the last decade has also been used in dementia care. The Snoezelen room is a plain room without adornment, with white or cream walls, ceiling and carpet. With the room light dimmed, multisensory equipment projects glowing colours through fibre-optics and tubes of water that results in moving bubbles. Pleasing nature scenes or abstract patterns are projected on the walls. Mirror balls resurrected from the disco era are slowly rotated to produce small coloured dots. Quiet, calming music is played in the background and aromatherapy might be used as well to stim-ulate the sense of smell. As a carer accompanies the dementing person, touch and communication are encouraged as they explore the various effects. Usually sessions are of about 30 minutes' duration and held twice weekly on a one-to-one basis.

Research into this therapy is very limited and it is unclear whether there are any benefits over and above what might accrue from an activity program. There are reports that some people show improvements in social behaviour and communication for up to a month after therapy has ended. Some individuals respond very well; however, others are unable to tolerate the environment and may become very distressed. There is insufficient evidence for the widespread use of this approach.[15]

Physical restraints

The use of physical restraints is unfortunately widespread in aged care facilities, with a recent survey in South Australia reporting that over one-quarter of residents were being restrained. Most restraints are used to prevent falls, although there is little evidence that they are effective for this purpose. Others are used to prevent wandering. The most commonly used restraints are the 'posy' that is worn as a type of vest and tied to a chair, the lap belt that is also tied to a chair, the tray table placed in front of a chair, and raised cot sides.[16]

There are numerous problems with restraints. Firstly, most restrained people become more agitated because they are uncom-fortable, and behavioural disturbances usually worsen. Secondly, some restraints are dangerous, particularly lap restraints, which have been known to strangle older people who slip down from the chair. Others may cause circulatory problems. Third, many are applied as a consequence of inadequate staffing levels rather than as an appropriate response to a clinical problem. This often has the corollary of meaning that staff inadequately monitor the restraints. Fourth, too often restraints are applied without obtaining appropriate consent.

There are some situations where restraints are appropriate; for example, an acutely sick dementing person who keeps pulling out catheters may need to be temporarily restrained; some agitated dementing people become calmer at meal times with a tray table in front of them.

SUMMARY

Psychosocial treatments for dementia are largely about assisting the dementing person and their carers to live with the disease with the best possible quality of life. This is very similar to the holistic approaches used in other chronic illnesses. By concentrating on abilities rather than disabilities and by providing an emotionally supportive environment, psychosocial treatments allow the dementing person to function at an optimal level.

CHAPTER 9

FAMILIES AND OTHER CARERS

DEMENTIA HAS AN ENORMOUS impact upon family and friends. Living with a person with dementia is often very stressful, particularly as the dementia progresses into the moderate and severe stages, and personality and behavioural changes become more apparent. Observing the gradual decline of a loved one from a competent individual to an incompetent dependent can be a harrowing experience. The demands upon the time and emotions of those providing care—the carers—can be huge. A famous book written about caregiving in the mid-1980s, by Peter Rabins and Nancy Mace, was entitled *The 36-Hour Day*. The title said it all for so many carers and it instantly became a bestseller worldwide.[1] However, caregiving is not all negative, and in this chapter I consider some of the positive aspects.

THE IMPACT OF EARLY DEMENTIA

Pre-diagnosis

In previous chapters I have described how the early symptoms of dementia may be non-specific and are often attributed to other causes. Depending on the type of symptoms that predominate, the early impact of dementia upon family and friends is quite variable. There is little doubt, however, that spouses and others living with the dementing person experience the greatest impact.

Jim and his 74-year-old wife Penny lived a quiet, happy life. Jim first noticed that Penny was becoming forgetful when she kept losing her house keys. Initially it was a source of humour, but after it had happened repeatedly over a six-month period, Jim became aware that Penny was also forgetting telephone conversations and visits to friends, and was leaving the stove on. Penny was also retreating from her previous standards of household cleanliness and seemed more reliant on Jim to help around the house. This didn't bother Jim too much and he just put the memory lapses down to age. But what did bother him was Penny's increasing reluctance to allow him to spend his usual hour or two with his mates at the club a few days a week. She became very anxious and fearful that something would happen while he was away. Jim couldn't understand the change, as this had been a lifelong habit that Penny had always been content about. It was Penny's anxiety and Jim's mounting frustration with the restrictions on his lifestyle that resulted in him taking Penny, upon the advice of his son, to their local doctor to discuss the problem. Their doctor quickly cottoned on to Penny's forgetfulness and that it was likely to be part of an early dementia, but it was the first time that Jim had considered that the forgetfulness and the anxiety were linked.

This case illustrates that it is often not memory changes that cause the greatest concern early on, particularly when the carer does not recognise the symptoms as being abnormal. The point when lifestyle changes are forced upon the carer is often the point when help is requested. These days, however, more and more people are becoming aware that memory changes may be due to dementia, and it is increasingly common for the spouse to become concerned at the earliest signs of memory decline and hence arrange an assessment. For children with widowed parents who live alone, the impact of early dementia in their parent can present them with a number of conflicts, as illustrated in the following case.

Rachel was an organised woman. Married to Tom, a professional with a busy career, and the mother of three teenage children, she needed to be organised to fit in her part-time job as a teacher. Her widowed mother, Rose, lived nearby and being the oldest daughter, Rachel had always felt obligated to her. Over a period of eighteen months Rachel became aware that her mother's faculties were failing. Previously completely independent, Rose now needed to be reminded to pay her bills and was unable to do her shopping by herself. Rachel naturally stepped in to help and, before she knew it, was doing all her mother's shopping, managing her finances and preparing many of her meals. It was not long before Rachel started to feel burdened by her various roles, particularly when her husband started to grumble that he wasn't seeing her. She also felt bitter towards her younger brother, who couldn't understand why she was concerned and was not making any effort to help. It was these pressures that led Rachel to seek help from the local Aged Care Assessment Team. Through them a dementia assessment was arranged and community support services organised. It was only at the family meeting during the assessment that Rachel's husband and brother finally started to recognise the extent of the problem and Rachel's need for support.

Facing the diagnosis

As I noted in Chapter 6, the dementia assessment process should provide family members with the opportunity to come to grips with the diagnosis and start planning for the future. Most family members will have realised that there was something seriously wrong long before the person with dementia realised it, but family members may also have greater difficulty in initially accepting the news. Possibly the prospect of living with a person with confirmed dementia is different to living with someone who is 'a bit forgetful'. The future may suddenly appear bleaker as worst fears are confirmed: 'How will I cope with looking after him/her?' The spouse may worry about the chances that the children will be at risk of dementia; the children may worry about themselves and their own children: 'Am I going to get dementia?' 'When do we have to start looking for a nursing home?' All of these and other concerns may crowd in.

Family concerns about the genetic risk posed to children and grandchildren are common. It should be remembered, as was discussed in Chapter 3, that with late-onset Alzheimer's disease there is a less than 10 per cent chance that a first-degree relative (child or sibling) will develop Alzheimer's disease before the age of 78, and for second-degree relatives such as grandchildren the risk probably drops to less than 5 per cent.[2] With early onset Alzheimer's disease the situation is quite different, as discussed below. Most other types of dementia have some degree of genetic influence, but there is less research data to provide families with accurate estimates of risk. In general, though, families can be largely reassured about their own risks of developing dementia.

Early management decisions

Many family members and persons with dementia are well aware of the 'new Alzheimer drugs' (cholinesterase inhibitors) and are keen to commence treatment. Imagine the disappointment that some families experience when they are told that their relative does have dementia, but it is not Alzheimer's disease and the new drugs are not proven to be suitable for use. Of course, as indicated in Chapter 7, Alzheimer's disease often coexists with other types of dementia, especially vascular dementia and dementia with Lewy bodies, and in these cases the cholinesterase inhibitors can frequently be reasonably prescribed under Australian PBS regulations. However, where it is quite clear that the type of dementia is definitely not Alzheimer's disease, there are no grounds under the PBS regulations for obtaining the subsidy. There are numerous case reports suggesting the cholinesterase inhibitors may benefit types of dementia as diverse as those associated with Parkinson's disease and multiple sclerosis, though the scientific strength of the research in these areas is weak. It is possible to have an unsubsidised trial of cholinesterase inhibitors in these circumstances, and some families elect to do so.

As far as possible, it is desirable that the dementing person chooses those family members they wish to participate in their decision making. Sometimes family conflicts or geographical separation (children interstate or overseas) prevent this from happening effectively, but there are often ways to get around difficulties. For example, I have found that email is an effective way for distantly located children to communicate with me (and other family members) about their parents. In general the types of early decisions that need to be made relate to financial management (enduring power of attorney, making a will), driving and possibly enduring guardianship, all described in detail in Chapter 12. All such decision making is assisted by family education about dementia in general, with specific information about the type of dementia which has been diagnosed. Usually there is no need to discuss the potential need for nursing home placement at this early stage, but some families do seek particular information.

I usually direct family members to the Alzheimer's Association, contactable either by phone or Internet, to get more information (see Appendices 1 and 2), and suggest they join the Association's carer support groups.

In early dementia it is desirable that families try to live as normally as possible. In many areas there will be no need to make major lifestyle changes. However, if the dementing person or the family have particular ambitions or plans to take a specific holiday trip or take up a new pastime, then it is 'now or never'. Meeting some ambitions may already be beyond the capacity of the dementing person, for example, undertaking a university course or an adventure expedition, but many other things are still quite achievable and most are desirable. Nostalgia trips to childhood and adolescent neighbourhoods are popular, particularly for migrants.

Issues in early onset dementia

When a person under 60 years of age develops dementia, the family impact can be devastating from a number of perspectives. The diagnosis of any serious, incurable illness is harder to deal with in a younger person than in old age, largely because such illnesses are 'out of phase' with what most of us expect to happen at that life stage. This is much more the case with dementia, not only due to its very nature, but also because it is very much a disease of old age. The life plans of the dementing person and their families are permanently disrupted.

Younger people with dementia are likely to be in the workforce, and usually the dementia will mean early retirement. Unless they have been contributing to a good superannuation scheme or have disability insurance, this often means a significant reduction in family income with all of its associated ramifications, including difficulties in meeting mortgage and debt repayments, and lifestyle changes. Where a spouse retires early to look after a dementing partner, there may be a similar effect.

It is also more likely that the dementing person will have children still at home. The effect of living with a dementing parent may be overwhelming, and there are some very moving testimonials written by school-age children.[3] To some extent, the degree to which children cope with the situation depends on how well the other parent is coping. But that is to oversimplify the situation. Even when the other parent is coping well, children need special attention to help them understand what is happening. The type of support a child needs varies with age, particularly in terms of how best to provide explanation. Fortunately the Alzheimer's Association has publications for children that can assist; the involvement of child and adolescent counselling services is usually helpful.[4]

Another difficult issue with early onset dementia is the increased likelihood that the dementia may be hereditary. As described in Chapters 3 and 4, some dementias in this age group may have a 50 per cent chance of being transmitted to offspring. This is particularly likely if there have been three or more first-degree family members with a dementia diagnosis. In these circumstances genetic counselling is advisable. Predictive genetic testing is possible, but there is at least a 30 per cent chance that no genetic mutation will be found. In the absence of any treatments to prevent the expression of the dementia if a mutation were found, most people do not want to know and the take-up for predictive testing is low.

Later in the course of dementia, if placement becomes a consideration, most families will find that there are few if any residential facilities that suit the younger person with dementia. Over half the residents in aged care facilities are aged 85 years and over, and a person in their 40s or 50s will usually feel out of place.[5] This difficulty can mean much unneeded added stress.

THE IMPACT OF MODERATE DEMENTIA

As described in Chapter 4, in the moderate stage of dementia the dementing person requires some level of assistance from other people to enable them to maintain their function in the community at a level as near as possible to the level they enjoyed before the onset of the dementia. It is often in this stage that carers begin to realise the full extent of the various demands upon their time. While the deteriorating memory function is a problem, it is usually not the main feature that impacts upon the carer. It is more often the personality and behavioural changes that cause the most concern, having the greatest effect on those carers who live with the dementing person, usually the spouse. During this stage of dementia, not only does it become very difficult for the dementing person to live independently, but it also becomes very difficult for the co-resident carer to have a life of his or her own.

What types of demands are placed upon the carer? The following examples give some indication.

Max had suffered from vascular dementia for three years. As his dementia worsened, he began to wake up regularly through the night. For a while his wife Doreen was able to settle him, and he would sleep fitfully for a few more hours. Eventually, he would regularly awaken at around 3 am, convinced that it was morning and time to go to work. No amount of persuasion from Doreen could convince him otherwise as he dressed and demanded his breakfast. To avoid conflict she would have to get up and pretend for an hour or so to help him go to work before she would be able to distract him by putting on the television.

Every few minutes Vicki would ask her husband Pete when they were going out to their daughter's home. He would reply as calmly as he could that they were leaving in two hours as she was still at work. After an hour he would start to get quite frustrated and decide to leave early. Once they were there, every few minutes Vicki would ask when they would be going home. This pattern recurred daily, to Pete's consternation.

Tony had always been a walker, a habit that didn't change as his dementia progressed. He would be out every morning for a couple of hours walking around the neighbourhood. His wife Karen was increasingly concerned about Tony's safety, particularly as he seemed so confused at home at the best of times and on the occasions when he was with her at the shops seemed oblivious to his surroundings. One morning he failed to return at his usual time and Karen was really worried. She searched the immediate neighbourhood without success. Five hours later the local police brought him home—he had been found wandering along the side of a motorway, obviously lost. To prevent this happening again, Karen decided it would be easier to walk with Tony every morning herself than trying to stop his lifelong habit.

Disrupted sleep patterns, repetitive questioning and wandering are just three examples of behaviours that place demands upon the carer's time and cause enormous strain or burden. Some of these behaviours require extra supervision from the carer, especially the sleep changes and wandering, increasing the demands on their time and requiring them to be vigilant even when they need time for themselves to relax. Some other types of behavioural and personality change, including aggressive outbursts and paranoid accusations, have a greater impact upon the actual relationship between the dementing person and carer and can threaten the well-being of the carer. (Examples of such situations appear in Chapter 4.) When the fundamental basis of a relationship is being undermined by such behaviours, even the most empathic, understanding and tolerant carer must eventually come to a breaking point. Fortunately, these behaviours are far from universal, and in many cases may improve with the medical and psychosocial strategies described in previous chapters. Probably the most important way of helping carers deal with these problems is through family education and support, as described later in this chapter.

Abuse of dementing people by carers

Occuring in a minority of cases, abuse of the dementing person by the carer is one of the negative consequences of caregiving that may emerge in this moderate stage of dementia. While elder abuse also occurs in the general population, persons with dementia are at increased risk. Most perpetrators of abuse live with the victim and deliver a significant amount of care. Carers who admit to abuse are more likely than non-abusers to have a history of mental illness and alcohol abuse. They are also more likely to report that they have been physically abused by the dementing person, often for many years before the dementia developed. It is generally accepted that there are basically two groups of abusive carers.[6]

The first group consists of bona fide carers who are under enormous stress and get caught up in a cycle of despair that engulfs them. These carers really need support and respite from their circumstances, as discussed later in this chapter and in Chapter 10. Usually, continued home care can continue once the issues that have provoked the crisis are addressed.

The second group has been labelled as 'pathological carers'; they perpetrate serious abuse as part of a lifestyle of violence, sociopathic behaviour and abuse of drugs and alcohol. In these cases other abusive behaviours, including sexual abuse and financial abuse, are more likely to happen. The only reasonable solution is protection of the dementing person, which generally means permanent separation from the carer. The dilemma here is that this often means placement into residential care, and the dementing person will frequently state a preference to remain at home, despite the abuse, to avoid placement. In Australia, the regional Aged Care Assessment Team (ACAT) is the main agency responsible for the investigation and management of elder abuse. Often the ACAT has to apply for a public guardian to be appointed to ensure that appropriate decisions are made on behalf of the dementing person (see Chapter 12).

THE IMPACT OF SEVERE DEMENTIA

In severe dementia, as described in Chapter 4, there is no semblance of independent function and maintenance at home usually requires 24-hour care from family, friends and community support services. This involves assistance with all basic activities of daily living—feeding, toileting, dressing, bathing and grooming. In addition, the behavioural changes previously described tend to persist, and will often worsen before there is a diminution as the dementia becomes more advanced. The following case typifies the impact upon the carer.

Adele was looking after her husband Philip, who had severe Alzheimer's disease. Her daily routine began around 6 am, when Philip awoke and noisily started to try to dress himself. Without her help he would usually put on his clothes inside out, or try to put his arms through his trouser legs, getting himself into a frustrated mess. Breakfast followed and of course she would have to monitor his feeding, make sure he got the cereal into his mouth, that his toast was cut and that his tea was not too hot. Then she would try to entice him to have a wash and allow her to shave him so that he would be ready to be picked up by the day centre bus at around 9.30 am. When he was at the day centre, two days a week, Adele would take the opportunity to do her shopping and have some time with friends. This was really the only time she had to relax apart from periods on the weekend when her daughter would help out. All other days she had to be with him full-time, as he could no longer be left alone for more than a few minutes. He had a tendency to wander and had got lost several times already. Fortunately Philip remained a placid man who could still show affection, even though his speech was now very limited. This helped Adele to keep going.

When physical ailments are also present, the burden upon the carer is amplified.

Richard had severe vascular dementia. He had just suffered another stroke and was now unable to walk without assistance. His memory was very poor and he was often disoriented. He wet the bed every night and needed assistance from his wife Cindy to shower and dress. Richard was a heavy man and Cindy quite petite; despite her best efforts and the assistance of community nurses, it was clear to all the health professionals involved that Cindy was unlikely to cope much longer. When advised to place her husband into a nursing home, Cindy vehemently refused. Intellectually, she understood that she was at the limits of her ability to look after Richard. Emotionally, she could not bear to part from her confidant. It was only when Richard had yet another stroke that the hospital geriatrician and social worker were able to convince her that placement was the best option.

It is usually during this stage of dementia that families have to grapple with the difficult task of placement; it might come earlier if the dementing person lives alone. This is often an emotionally distressing period for carers, especially if they have been determined to look after the dementing person at home until they die. The reality is that very few carers are able to achieve this ambition; 24-hour care is enormously difficult to provide over a period of some years, even with the involvement of community services. Those fortunate enough to be able to self-fund 24-hour personal care assistants to take the load off their shoulders are more likely to achieve it but the costs are prohibitive. I cover issues related to community services and residential care in Chapters 10 and 11.

The other major issue confronting carers by this stage of dementia is the grieving process. Anticipatory grief, in which a person begins to grieve before the death of a loved one, is particularly common in severe dementia due to the premature loss of many of the personal attributes upon which the relationship was based, otherwise known as the 'self', but it is also a significant factor contributing to carer stress earlier in the dementia. When your loved one no longer recognises you, is generally incoherent and lives in a nursing home; it is little wonder that it seems as if they have died. For some carers, the grieving process may be virtually completed before the dementing person's death. This often results in cessation of visits to the nursing home and irritation at being asked to remain involved. For other carers, anticipatory grief has the effect of drawing out the grieving process for a much longer period than with many other terminal illnesses, resulting in a chronic period of heightened emotions that may take years to resolve even after the death. Jonathan Franzen, in his novel *The Corrections*, writes about the death of his father from Alzheimer's disease. He comments on how he had been mourning his father for years before he died. He also notes that even in the advanced stage of dementia, when his father could no longer recognise him, he felt compelled to look for meaning in his father's existence and was surprised that he kept finding it.[7] This search for meaning is an experience common to many carers.

GENDER DIFFERENCES

In general, female carers seem to suffer higher levels of distress than male carers. There are many theories about this. Certainly, women in our society are more likely to be thrust into the caregiving role than men and may have less choice about it. Female carers are also more likely to be 'hands-on', that is, they tend to do everything themselves rather than delegate to others. Male carers tend to have more of a 'managerial' style that allows them to distance themselves from the stressful situation to some degree by delegating tasks.[8]

Another factor contributing to the differential experience of stress relates to the psychological development and social roles fulfilled by men and women at different stages of the life cycle.[9] Historically, women have tended to have a nurturing and caring role in their early to mid-adult life through child rearing. When the children grew up, women tended to pursue their personal development through a delayed career or other interests. A return to a primary nurturing and caring role may not fit in with many women's later life plans. In contrast, men during their early to mid-adult life have tended to be in the workforce and have not had much of a nurturing role. As they age, men's psychological development turns to a more nurturing role, best exemplified by the grandfather who spends more time with his grandchildren than he ever did with his children. Thus, for some older men the nurturing role of caregiving may be more in keeping with their personal development than it is for some older women.

FAMILY EDUCATION AND SUPPORT

Education about dementia is an essential component of helping families live with a dementing person. At its simplest level, initial education may involve the provision of information about the type of dementia, its course, what to expect, what plans to make and the treatments available. This might be delivered at the time of diagnosis by the assessment team, or by books, brochures and the Internet. Information about specific problems such as behavioural changes may be needed as the circumstances arise. But knowledge alone is usually insufficient, as has been demonstrated in a few studies.

In one of the major studies in this field in the late 1980s, Professor Henry Brodaty, with Meredith Gresham, developed a carers' training program at Prince Henry Hospital in Sydney. The structured, intensive ten-day residential program involved a mix of education, skills training and stress management as a package delivered early in the course of dementia. After the period of initial training, ongoing emotional support was provided in groups and by teleconferences. The design of the study compared three randomly allocated groups. The first group of carers received the training program immediately; the second group was placed on a 'wait list' and received the program six months later; the third group received ten days of respite care. During the period of the program, each of the dementing persons received a ten-day structured memory training and activity program. The study found that carer stress was significantly lower in those carers who received training. Just as importantly, the benefits persisted. The earlier in the course of dementia that a carer received the training package, the greater the perceived benefit. One of the surprising findings was that benefits appeared to persist for up to eight years. Nursing home placement was delayed and, quite unexpectedly, survival of the person with dementia was longer. This survival was not simply related to delays in nursing home placement and could not be explained by any particular features of the person's dementia.[10]

There is now a growing body of research worldwide that has demonstrated the benefits of family education and support, though attempts to identify the critical components of the various training programs used around the world have not been very successful. Further, training programs do not suit everybody. There is some evidence that suggests that while early intervention is important, carers also need to be ready for the intervention. If the family member feels in control of the situation and does not feel under any stress, they may not feel that attending a program is of much use at that time and would rather wait until they feel it is necessary. In other cases, readiness to undertake training may be related more to the carer's psychological preparedness to deal with the problem than to any sense of being in control. Carers who are feeling stressed and are looking for answers probably obtain the greatest benefit from this type of program. The Alzheimer's Association has developed a 'Living with memory loss' program that involves both the carer and the person with early dementia, in a course of separate group sessions.

Most research in the field of caring has focused on the primary carer and paid little attention to other family members. This has been particularly the case when other family members live interstate or overseas. There is mounting evidence, however, that the involvement of as many family members as possible in the education and support process is beneficial. Frequently the designated primary carer, for example the spouse, can only effectively fulfil that role with the active support of other family members such as the children or siblings. Including the other family members within the educational and support program makes it more likely that the primary carer will receive support. Individuals within the one family, however, may have different degrees of preparedness and willingness to participate in carer training programs and may not wish to participate all at the same time. Often, however, important issues arise that can only be effectively dealt with in the family group, especially when individual family members have differing opinions about what should happen. Conflict most commonly emerges during the period when institutional care is being considered. Other issues that may be the basis for conflict include financial management and the use of medications.

ALZHEIMER'S ASSOCIATION

Many services involved in dementia care in Australia run education and support groups for dementia carers in various formats. In the main, funding for these types of programs has been allocated to the Alzheimer's Association, which has developed an impressive array of services for carers. In Chapter 4 I described how 30 years ago the realisation that 'senile dementia' was in fact the same as Alzheimer's disease led to a massive increase in research into the fundamental causes of Alzheimer's disease. Probably the second major influence in the field of dementia was the emergence about 20 years ago, in the early 1980s, of consumer-based organisations in different Australian states that evolved into the Alzheimer's Association. Initially set up to provide support to dementia carers during an era when little was available in the community, the Alzheimer's Association is now the peak consumer group representing both dementia carers and, in more recent years, people with dementia. Importantly, the organisation embraces health professionals and uses these partnerships to provide its members with the latest information on the research front. It is part of a worldwide network of Alzheimer associations coordinated through Alzheimer's Disease International.

In Australia, the critical role that the Alzheimer's Association has played in lobbying governments to improve services for dementia care cannot be overemphasised. Politicians listen more to consumers than to health professionals about service requirements, and the cogent arguments and submissions provided by the Alzheimer's Association has seen funding flow to a range of projects, including 24-hour telephone helplines for carers, carer education programs for various ethnic groups, programs for people with early dementia, carer respite programs and various carer support groups. Most services involved with dementia care in Australia have developed strong links with their local Alzheimer's Association. In many cases they supply the group leaders for their local Alzheimer's Association carer support groups. Details of how to contact the Alzheimer's Association are listed in Appendices 1 and 2.

POSITIVE ASPECTS OF CAREGIVING

Caregiving should not be characterised only by its negative attributes. Many carers report heightened feelings of love and affection for the dementing person arising from the caregiving experience. The relationship may become closer through the sharing of life experiences that might not have otherwise occurred. There is often a sense of reciprocation in which carers feel they are repaying an emotional debt to the dementing person. This is particularly the case with adult children who feel their parent has made sacrifices for them. There is also an element of this with many male carers.

When Michael's wife Sarah was diagnosed with Alzheimer's disease just short of her 75th birthday, Michael was determined that she would be well looked after. Married for 55 years, they had had a number of ups and downs but they had always pulled through. Michael felt that Sarah deserved his care and attention; for one thing, he had never forgotten the support she provided when he returned injured after the Second World War. In more recent years she had helped him pull through a cancer scare. Michael was diligent in finding out about the community services available to assist dementia carers, but reasoned that he would only call on them when needed. Despite having to learn how to cook, and forever having difficulty with the ironing, Michael seemed to thrive. He made use of the dementia day care centre each week and found the time that this availed him to be sufficient to get his chores done. He kept in touch with his mates and was fortunate that he could still get out to the club for a few hours each week with Sarah. She enjoyed this and Michael was constantly surprised by how 'normally' she could behave.

Caregiving is full of challenges and for many carers it brings an opportunity to broaden their life experiences, albeit not necessarily in the way they had planned. Personal growth may be attained through the mastery of new skills and better self-awareness. For example, women commonly have to learn about financial management and men often have to learn about household management, both of which can bring a sense of achievement. In relationships where the carer has been subservient to a domineering partner, increased personal autonomy may occur as the carers gradually gain confidence to more fully express themselves.

SUMMARY

Dementia has a major impact upon the dementing person's family and friends. Family carers take up the brunt of the burden of care in mild and moderate dementia; by the time the dementia is severe, however, most have reached the end of their tether and have had to place the dementing person into residential care. Despite this, many carers report positive experiences from care-giving. The Alzheimer's Association has developed as the primary consumer organisation for support of carers and, in recent years, for persons with dementia.

CHAPTER 10

COMMUNITY CARE SERVICES

M OST PEOPLE WITH A terminal illness would probably prefer to live at home until they die. Most families would probably prefer to look after their disabled relatives for as long as possible at home. However, because dementia is such a slowly progressive condition, by comparison with illnesses such as cancer, the time frame over which care needs to be provided is very long. Without a strong community care system, most families and other carers are hamstrung in their efforts to look after the person with dementia at home.

HISTORY OF COMMUNITY CARE IN AUSTRALIA

Australia has earned a good reputation in international circles for its high quality community care services. That hasn't always been the case, however. In the early 1980s, few community-based services were available for dementia care. Various forms of respite care and community support that are now routinely available did not exist. Most health services provided no dementia-specific services. There was no routine dementia assessment. Family carers struggled along with limited support from friends, GPs and specialists until they could cope no longer and had to place their loved ones into an institution, usually either a psychiatric hospital or a nursing home. There was minimal community recognition of their plight, few places to get information about dementia (even the local GP was unlikely to know much) and no carer allowances or pensions from the government to help defray the economic burden of care.[1]

In the early 1980s serious questions began to be asked about the direction of Australian Commonwealth Government funding for aged care. With the ageing population, government funding for nursing homes was spiralling out of control while very little was being invested into community services to support older people in their own homes. In other words, the service structures were designed to look after people in institutions rather than in the community. The 1986 landmark Nursing Home and Hostel Review set the ball into motion for change with an Aged Care Reform Strategy.[2] Apart from setting up the forerunners of the current Aged Care Assessment Teams (ACATs), which have the responsibility of determining the eligibility of people for government-subsidised institutional care and community services based upon their level of disability, it also set limits on the number of nursing home beds that were to be funded, redirecting the funding to community-based services.

The four basic philosophical tenets underpinning the review were:

1. to provide support to older and disabled people in their own homes;
2. to provide residential services to older and disabled people only where their needs are not appropriately met by other support systems;
3. for services to have a rehabilitation focus to restore function in a manner that develops and enhances personal freedom and independent functioning; and
4. to recognise that for many older and disabled people, less supported residential services or community-based support services will be a possible and desirable outcome.[3]

Dementia was recognised in the review as a major cause of disability that required institutional care, and funding for dementia-specific community services started to flow in the late 1980s. Three types of dementia-specific community services can be identified:

- Dementia assessment services to ensure accurate diagnoses are being made and reversible causes treated;
- Disability support services to allow disabled dementing people to live in their homes for as long as possible;

• Carer support services to reduce carer stress and hence allow carers to cope with community care for longer periods.

In 1990, a Mid Term Review of the Aged Care Reform Strategy was commenced, with dementia care being one of the main areas addressed. Out of the recommendations of this review came the National Action Plan for Dementia Care, launched in 1992. The plan covered seven elements—assessment, services for people with dementia, services for carers, quality of care, community awareness, research, and policy and planning.[4]

Over the last fifteen years, the Australian community-care sector has grown enormously in each of these areas, with 41 demonstration projects being piloted, some of which have evolved into standard service delivery. Many are based on models from other countries adapted to Australian conditions. It is difficult to keep up with all the changes in community services and indeed a number of problems have emerged. In 2001, Aged and Community Services Australia released a discussion paper on community care that highlighted four areas of concern— problems with service coordination and integration; inflexibility in community service program rules for eligibility that can result in gaps; rivalry between the Commonwealth and the States over funding and administration; and uncoordinated planning of serv- ices. In essence, the whole system has become too bureaucratic and is confusing for carers, care recipients and health professionals alike.[5]

One way to find out what is available in your local area is to contact a Commonwealth Carelink Centre, either by phone or in person (see Appendix 1). These centres provide a point of contact for information about local community and health services. In the rest of this chapter I describe the various types of community services available in Australia (see Table 10.1) and how to access them.

AGED CARE ASSESSMENT PROGRAM

What is the Aged Care Assessment Program?

This is the program under which the Australian Government provides grants to State and Territory Governments specifically to

Table 10.1 Types of community services available in Australia

Service type	What they do
Aged Care Assessment Program	This is a nationwide network system of Aged Care Assessment Teams (ACATs) that provides comprehensive multidisciplinary assessment of older and disabled people in order to facilitate access to appropriate available community services. Most ACATs have geriatricians on their teams.
Home and Community Care (HACC) Program	Provides support for older people, people with disabilities and their carers through services such as home care, meals, transport, respite, nursing, personal care and home maintenance.
Community Options Programs	Brokerage-style services in which case coordinators can put together packages of care from different service providers for people with complex needs.
Community Aged Care Packages (CACPs)	Offer an integrated package of services as an alternative to residential care, which may include home help, laundry, shopping, and assistance with meals, medication monitoring, social support and bathing.
Carer Services	Includes Commonwealth Carer Resource Centres, Commonwealth Carer Respite Centres, residential and day respite care, carer allowances and payments.
Aged Care Psychiatry (Psychogeriatric) Services	Services that treat older people with mental health problems. In dementia care, their main involvement occurs if there are significant behavioural and psychological symptoms complicating the dementia.
Innovative Community Services	These services are being piloted around Australia and include Extended Aged Care at Home Packages, Innovative Care Dementia Services, and Hospital in the Home services.

operate ACATs (known as Aged Care Assessment Services in Victoria). It is a nationwide network system for the comprehensive assessment of older and disabled people in order to facilitate access to appropriate available community services. The organisation of ACATs varies from State to State but they are all based on geographical catchment areas. Some are co-located with other aged care services, others are stand-alone services. Some provide only assessment services, others provide continuing care as well. ACATs also determine eligibility for Commonwealth-subsidised residential aged care, Community Aged Care Packages (CACPs) and some flexible care services. In other words they are gatekeepers, and as such operate under Commonwealth regulatory guidelines when making their decisions.[6]

One of the key objectives of the program is to ensure that people with dementia have equitable access to ACATs. In New South Wales, about 26 per cent of ACAT referrals have dementia so this objective is usually achieved. Other important objectives include:

- Prevention of premature or inappropriate admissions to aged care facilities;
- Comprehensive assessment that encompasses the restorative, physical, medical, psychological, cultural and social dimensions of care need;
- Involvement of clients, their carers and other service providers in the assessment and care planning process;
- Improvement of the appropriateness and range of care services available through the promotion of coordinated services. This requires the ACATs to establish links with other services, GPs and hospitals.[7]

When do you contact your local ACAT?

How early in the course of dementia a local ACAT is contacted will vary depending on location and individual circumstances. It is probably best to discuss individual circumstances with a GP. In some parts of Australia, particularly rural and regional areas, ACATs are the primary setting for initial dementia assessment and the GP or another health professional might make a referral for this to occur. There may not be any other need for community services at this point.

Probably the two main reasons to contact the ACAT are to access community services, which may include respite care, CACPs and Home and Community Care (HACC) services, and to arrange assessment for placement into a residential aged care facility. This latter assessment is recorded on the Aged Care Client Record. Information about how to contact your local ACAT is found in Appendices 1 and 2.

Who performs the assessment on the ACAT?

ACATs are multidisciplinary teams capable of making thorough assessments of their clients' needs. Most ACATs include a geriatrician or physician, registered nurses, social workers, physiotherapists and occupational therapists. Access to other disciplines such as psychogeriatricians, psychologists, speech therapists, podiatrists and dietitians is often available on a sessional basis. It is usual practice following the referral that a case manager from the team is allocated, based on the information obtained from the referring person. In many teams dementia care workers—usually registered nurses or social workers—make the initial assessment.

What does an ACAT assessment involve?

At the time of referral, cases are allocated a priority category based upon the urgency of need. There are three categories: within 48 hours (for example, where there is risk of immediate harm); three to fourteen days (for example, where there is no immediate risk of harm but current level of care doesn't meet the person's needs); and over fourteen days (for example, where respite care is planned). The type of assessment performed depends on the individual case. New referrals require a thorough, holistic, independent assessment from the case manager that covers the needs of the client and the carer, the client's medical history, mental functioning physical functioning, and living conditions. The involvement of other disciplines is arranged according to need. For example, if the referred patient has a history consistent with dementia but has not had a dementia assessment, a formal assessment involving a geriatrician or psychogeriatrician is usually arranged. Multidisciplinary assessment can be achieved through case conferencing, joint assessments, follow-up visits and cross-referral to other services such as aged care psychiatry services. Case-conferencing is often used for complex or difficult assessments. In all cases the case manager will have to complete a Minimum Data Set that includes all this information along with their recommendations for services. Aggregated data (without identifying information) from the Minimum Data Set are forwarded every three months to an Evaluation Unit that monitors ACAT activities in order to determine whether the program is adequately addressing client need.[8]

What are the potential outcomes of an ACAT assessment?

The assessment process should result in a care plan formulated to take account of input from the case manager, client and carers. This may involve further assessments by other health professionals, referrals to community care services (as described later in the chapter) and completion of an Aged Care Client Record that authorises access to CACPs and residential care along with the level of care required (high or low). ACAT approvals are valid for twelve months, though reassessments will be required in circumstances such as transfer from low to high care and from respite to permanent residential care. When the ACAT is part of a broader aged care service, it is likely that some level of ongoing support will be provided until the recommended actions have commenced. Occasionally, the client or carer does not agree with the assessment outcome and in those circumstances there is a right of appeal.[9]

HOME AND COMMUNITY CARE (HACC) PROGRAM

HACC is a joint Commonwealth/State cost-shared program that provides support for older people, people with disabilities and their carers. About 10 per cent of Australians over 70 years of age receive HACC services. The program assists people who are at risk of premature or inappropriate long-term residential care, and their carers, and aims to enhance their independence and quality of life.[10] There is no need for an ACAT assessment to access HACC services, though many referrals come from ACATs. Self-referral is possible, though in most cases referrals are organised by GPs, hospitals, aged care and aged care psychiatry services. HACC provides a wide range of services that includes:

- home help, including housework, laundry and shopping;
- home maintenance or modification;
- personal care, such as toileting, bathing, dressing and feeding;
- home nursing;
- meal preparation and home-delivered meals;
- physiotherapy, podiatry, occupational therapy and speech therapy;
- respite care, including day care and in-home respite;
- transport.

There are numerous government and non-government agencies providing HACC services. Most of the community nursing, podiatry, physiotherapy, occupational therapy and speech therapy services are located within community health and aged care services run by the State Governments, Territory Governments and local governments. These may be co-located with ACATs. Services such as meals, home help and community transport tend to be run by non-government agencies such as charitable organisations, church organisations and other community groups. All agencies are bound by a set of national service standards that emphasise issues such as the importance of access, accurate assessment, involvement of consumers in care planning, adequate documentation, monitoring of outcomes, training and supervision of staff, and relationships with ACATs. These standards are designed to ensure that people who have more complex needs and require a more comprehensive assessment are identified early and appropriate action taken.[11] While service fees are not mandatory, most HACC services levy a small charge.

An HACC service not available in all areas, and known as Community Options Programs (or Linkages in Victoria), is a brokerage-style service in which case coordinators can put together packages of care from different service providers for people with complex needs. The amount of care provided is not specifically limited. If the care recipient can afford to pay for extra services, the coordinator can often arrange it if it is locally available.

CARER SERVICES

There are many types of services available for carers. The Commonwealth Carer Resource Centres (see Appendix 1) are handy single points at which to obtain advice and information about services, support and publications available for carers. Carer Information Packs, which include information about financial, legal, safety, health and self-care matters, as well as a relaxation CD/tape and an Emergency Care Plan, are available at these centres. These are also available from the Carers Association.[12] Of course, many services for carers also benefit the care recipient as well so it is rather an artificial distinction.

Respite care

Respite care is particularly important for both people with dementia and their carers. A number of types of respite care are available, ranging in duration from a few hours to a few months. Each local area of Australia has a Commonwealth Carer Respite Centre that coordinates access to respite services and provides advice to carers about respite (see Appendices 1 and 2).[13]

Probably the most frequently utilised form of respite care is dementia day care. Usually this involves the dementing person being picked up by bus between 9 and 10 am to spend about four or five hours in a day centre before being returned home between 3 and 4 pm. Day care benefits the dementing person through the social and diversional activities provided. It benefits the carer by allowing a much-needed break. There may be a period of adjustment when the dementing person first goes to the day centre. They may need a lot of persuasion to go there initially, but this reluctance usually settles quickly. Sometimes the carer may need to accompany them for the first few times.

Some dementing people absolutely refuse to leave their homes, and a co-resident carer may well feel trapped. In these circumstances in-home respite, where a community worker stays at home with the dementing person while the carer goes out, might work. This type of respite is also useful for a non-English speaking person when the community worker speaks their language. Sometimes overnight respite can be arranged.

Residential respite care is usually provided in an aged care facility. In most cases this is alongside permanent residents, though there are some facilities that specialise in respite care. There is a nine-week annual entitlement to residential respite care, which in some circumstances can be extended to twelve weeks. All residential respite care must be approved through an ACAT assessment. Planned residential respite usually covers circumstances such as allowing the carer to have a holiday, to undergo a non-urgent surgical procedure, or just simply a rest. Some carers take three or four respite breaks per year for two or three weeks at a time. There have been complaints that in some areas planned respite is difficult to arrange at times suitable to the carer, and that some facilities won't give booking confirmations until close to the date, which is very stressful to a carer trying to make specific personal arrangements. Emergency respite can sometimes be arranged if the carer has an acute illness or crisis that prevents them from looking after the dementing person, but is unfortunately very difficult to access.[14]

There is some debate in the literature about whether residential respite care may cause harm to the dementing person by increasing their confusion and agitation, along with the likelihood that psychotropic medication will be required to settle them. Certainly there are individual cases where the period of residential respite becomes quite traumatic both for the dementing person and the carer. Occasions where the carer is summoned in the middle of the night to take home an extremely agitated person can be very disturbing for all concerned. In most cases, however, there are few dramas outside the expected settling-in period of the first few days.

For some carers, residential respite care is a prelude to permanent placement. During the course of the respite admission a carer may indicate that they are unable to take the dementing person home again. In my experience this is most likely to happen with a very stressed carer who has been putting off taking a period of respite for a long time and, having had a taste of life as a non-carer, suddenly realises that they just can't deal with the situation any longer. In these circumstances every effort is usually made to accommodate the situation by finding a permanent long-term placement, often in the same facility.

Respite residents are charged a flat fee that is not means tested; it is set at the standard pensioner contribution to residential care irrespective of whether or not they are pensioners (this was up to $25.73 daily in March 2003). Usually a booking fee is paid when respite admissions are arranged.[15]

Carer Allowance and Carer Payment

In Australia, the Commonwealth Government provides two types of payments to carers. The Carer Allowance is for co-resident carers who provide full-time care to a person with a severe medical condition or disability, such as dementia. There are criteria of disability as measured on the Adult Disability Assessment Tool administered by staff from Centrelink. The payment is non-taxable and is not subjected to either an assets or income test. In March 2003, the payment was $87.70 per fortnight.[16]

The Carer Payment (formerly the Carers Pension) is for carers who provide full-time care to a person with a severe medical condition or disability, such as dementia, with similar levels of disability as required for the Carer Allowance. This does not need to be co-resident care. Often the carer has had to give up their regular employment to provide the care. The Carer Payment is not available to carers in receipt of another pension. As with other pensions, the amount a carer is eligible to receive is affected by income and assets. Rent assistance may be available. In March 2003, the maximum single payment was $440.30 per fortnight and for a couple $367.50 each per fortnight.[17]

COMMUNITY AGED CARE PACKAGES (CACPs)

CACPs, introduced in 1992, are community care services tailored to meet the needs of individuals. They offer an integrated package of services, which may include home help, laundry, shopping, and assistance with meals, medication monitoring, social support and bathing. The services are coordinated through one agency to make it easier for the clients. Usually a care coordinator from the agency puts together the individualised package of care in consultation with the care recipient and their informal carer. CACPs are designed as an alternative to residential care, so access to them is based on an initial ACAT assessment determining the appropriate level of need. As CACPs are an alternative to residential care, only care recipients with complex needs are likely to meet the guidelines. Although the amount of care available through an individual package is not specified, on average around six hours of care per week is provided.

CACPs are provided by a range of non-government organisations which receive Commonwealth funding for a specific number of packages in a defined geographical region. In March 2003, the Commonwealth subsidy was $30.73 per day. Care recipients are charged a fee for the service, with those on the basic pension paying no more than 17.5 per cent of that pension ($5.29 per day in May 2003). Care recipients on a higher income may be asked to pay additional fees, but this is limited to 50 per cent of any income that exceeds the full pension rate. However, the Commonwealth Department of Health and Ageing states that no one will be denied a service through inability to pay.[18]

CACPs have been one of the more successful community care initiatives. Although by July 2001 there were 24 630 CACPs approved Australia-wide,[19] in my experience there is usually a shortfall in availability. The flexibility and range of the services offered often means that a dementing person can be managed at home when in the past the only reasonable alternative would have been placement, especially where that person lived alone. They are particularly effective for people from minority ethnic groups who do not speak English because particular attention can be paid to their dietary needs and case workers from that cultural background can be obtained, as can be seen in the following case.

Antonia was an 83-year-old, single, non-English speaking woman of Greek descent who had lived alone since her sister died some years earlier. Gradually over a period of some years her niece noted that she had become increasingly forgetful, suspicious and lonely. She would regularly lose her keys and her purse and accuse others of taking them. Her home was neglected, as was her personal hygiene. She wore the same filthy dress every day. Her diet was poor and she had lost around 10 kg over the previous few years. Following an ACAT assessment, a CACP package organised through the local Greek welfare service was commenced. The package involved regular visits from a Greek-speaking woman who did some of the housework and encouraged Antonia to bathe and change her clothes a few times per week. She could also assist in preparing the occasional Greek meal that supplemented regular Meals on Wheels. Antonia was also taken out to a Greek social club each week and she really enjoyed the company. Over some

> months she became much happier and put on some weight, though she still remained suspicious of the neighbours.

AGED CARE PSYCHIATRY (PSYCHOGERIATRIC OR MENTAL HEALTH FOR OLDER PEOPLE) SERVICES

These are State and Territory government services that treat older people with mental health problems in the community. In dementia care, their main involvement occurs where there are significant behavioural and psychological symptoms complicating the dementia. This is very important because of the high likelihood that if the symptoms continue unchecked, the dementing person may be prematurely placed in residential care. Apart from providing specialist treatment, aged care psychiatry services usually provide short to medium term support for carers, including some education about dealing with the problem. There is good evidence that when intensive case management is provided to persons with dementia and their carers, carer stress is reduced alongside improvements in function, socialisation and risk for the dementing person.[20] Sometimes brief hospital admission to an acute aged care psychiatry unit is necessary if the symptoms are severe.

Unfortunately, these services are unevenly provided around Australia. Some States, such as Victoria, have very comprehensive, well-funded and resourced services. Other States, such as New South Wales, are poorly funded and resourced. This means that unlike the Commonwealth-funded community services there is enormous variability with regards to availability. There is also variability in terms of service location, even within States. Some are co-located with other mental health services, others with aged care services, while others are stand alone. Probably the best place to get information about the service in a particular area would be through the local ACAT.

INNOVATIVE COMMUNITY SERVICES

A number of community care initiatives are in various stages of being piloted around Australia to determine whether they are potentially useful in a broader context. These are generally designed to be flexible and innovative in their attempts to improve the capacity to look after disabled and unwell older people at home. Some are designed to delay entry to residential care, others are designed to avoid hospital admissions or to allow earlier discharge from hospital.

Extended Aged Care at Home (EACH) Packages

This is a pilot program to see if it is feasible to provide the equivalent of high-level residential care at home. Ten centres across Australia are participating. The EACH packages offer older people the opportunity to be cared for at home instead of in residential care, and are probably better suited to the physically disabled than to persons with dementia. However, the program has yet to be formally evaluated to determine its financial viability, effectiveness and quality of care.[21]

Innovative Care Dementia Services

This new pilot program is not a specific form of community or residential dementia care but rather a flexible approach to improve the range of service options for people with dementia not well catered for by existing services. This might include dementing people living alone or with special needs that hinder service delivery. Currently expressions of interest are being taken for proposals.

Hospital in the Home programs

Numerous programs that have been piloted around the country aim to reduce the need for hospital care for physically unwell older people by providing a geriatric outreach service into the older person's home. The outreach service usually includes a geriatrician, nurses, physiotherapists and social workers who work in collaboration with the GP. The types of problems these services are particularly suited to treat include respiratory, urinary and skin infections, mild cardiac problems and soft tissue injuries after a fall. This might be initiated in the person's home following a GP referral; after an assessment in the local emergency department; or following a brief admission to hospital to facilitate early discharge. For people with dementia, hospital admission can be extremely traumatic with increased confusion and behavioural problems due to the illness and new environment. Home-based care can often reduce these complications and improve the outcome.

The future of community care in Australia

In August 2002, a coalition of nine professional bodies that included the Alzheimer's Association, Aged and Community Services Australia and the Australian Society for Geriatric Medicine released a discussion paper on a 'Vision for Community Care'. The stated vision was that 'community care of the future will support lifestyle choices to enable people who need support and their carers to live in their own community'.[22] This vision would involve 'seamless' service delivery in which the mechanism of obtaining services, particularly as care recipients' needs changed, would be largely invisible to the care recipient and have minimal bureaucracy. The philosophy of care emphasises greater flexibility in service delivery to meet the needs of individual care recipients in a tailored way, which is really an extension of what has been evolving over the last fifteen years. Moreover, the discussion paper envisaged that community care in the future should better recognise the knowledge, skills and capacities of care recipients, rather than concentrating on their deficits. Apart from less bureaucracy and overlapping, repetitive assessments, better linkages between health professionals in various settings would be required along with a single electronic health record with clear and stringent privacy safeguards. This would be aided by a single funding system with only one level of government being responsible for all community care that would incorporate all existing programs and interfaces with general practice and acute hospitals to promote better coordinated care. Other non-government sources of funding will probably be needed as well.

This seems an admirable vision, with the main stumbling block likely to be the removal of two levels of government from community care administration. I find it hard to imagine any level of government being agreeable to such a proposition, no matter how sensible it might appear to be.

Summary

Community services are particularly important in supporting dementing people and their carers at home. There is a broad range of services available in Australia focusing on providing accurate assessments, minimising the effects of disability, providing support to carers and determining eligibility to residential care. These processes of assessment are often confusing for health professionals and carers alike. The current trend in community services is to increase flexibility in care provision through innovative strategies.

CHAPTER 11

RESIDENTIAL CARE

MOST PEOPLE WITH DEMENTIA will be placed into residential care in the moderate–severe stage of their illness, despite the best efforts of carers and community services to support them at home. Carer stress is one of the major factors leading to the breakdown of community care, and this in turn is often related to the behavioural aspects of the dementia. Other factors include the demands of physical care, the health of the carer and the availability of community support. If the dementing person lives alone, placement is likely to come sooner, as it is very difficult to provide overnight supervision in a community setting. In this chapter I cover:

- the preparation required for entering residential care;
- the basic requirements of good residential care;
- the different types of residential care for dementia;
- the residential care system in Australia.

WHY DOES PLACEMENT INTO RESIDENTIAL CARE OCCUR?

Placement in many circumstances occurs because insufficient professional and non-professional community support is available to alleviate the pressure on carers or to look after a single dementing person in their own home. The reason behind insufficient community support is principally economic. Although residential care is very expensive, the cost of providing safe, quality, home-based care to people with severe dementia is even more expensive. Most people with severe dementia require 24-hour supervision and it is often the overnight care that is the stumbling block. The cost of community services that can provide this level of supervision is huge. Some wealthy people are able to afford it but the average person cannot. Residential care in this situation is really an economic solution to a difficult problem. This doesn't mean that we shouldn't be trying to further increase the community services that are available. At this stage, as implied from the pilot schemes described in the previous chapter, the actual point at which community service provision becomes economically unviable for quality care has yet to be determined. However, it should also be recognised that for some carers no amount of extra support will ever allow them to cope with the dementing person at home.

PREPARATION REQUIRED FOR ENTERING RESIDENTIAL CARE

Placement into a residential aged care facility is often a very stressful process for carers and the dementing person. Very few dementing people will go by choice. In my experience, the majority of older people who are keen to go into residential care are clinically depressed and feel that they are an unwanted burden on their family. Others seem agreeable to the placement and don't make a fuss, but usually they are quietly unhappy about it. Some will be vocally adamant that they will not go into 'a home'; at times a guardianship order will be required to provide legal authority for the placement against the dementing person's wishes (see Chapter 12 for more detail).

Some steps can be taken in an attempt to minimise the stress for carers and sometimes for the dementing person. Carers are advised to plan ahead from a reasonably early point in the dementing process by finding out about the various facilities in their area. All facilities are prepared to show people around, though usually by appointment. Usually it is just the carers who have a look, but occasionally an insightful dementing person may wish to participate in the decision making. Some facilities allow names to be placed on a waiting list even when there is no immediate plan for placement, but most request that there be a valid ACAT assessment (see Chapter 10) before doing so. I don't think there is much point in putting a person's name on a waiting list unless there seems to be a likelihood of placement within a year.

As described in the previous chapter, in Australia it is essential to obtain an assessment from an ACAT to determine the dementing person's eligibility for residential care. There are basic criteria of day-to-day function that determine whether a person is disabled enough for residential care and the type of care required. All persons with moderate dementia would be disabled enough to qualify for residential care, but this doesn't mean that they need to be placed because carers and community services are able to support many at home.[1]

How do you choose the 'best' facility? This is very difficult and often local availability is the main factor. If the dementing person is from a non-English speaking background, and particularly if they speak little English or have very strong religious or cultural beliefs, a facility that specifically caters for these needs is advisable. As there are relatively few such facilities, this may well mean that families will have to travel a significant distance to visit the dementing person.

Otherwise choice should be guided by three factors—facility condition and design, staff attitudes and knowledge, and the particular needs of the dementing person. These are all covered later in this chapter. Advice from the health professionals involved in the care of the dementing person (GP, community nurse, geriatrician, psychogeriatrician) should assist in the process. Sometimes a particular facility might appear excellent, but the health professionals may advise that it does not meet the dementing person's needs. If it is very important to the dementing person or the carer to maintain their long-term GP, check which facilities they visit. Quite often a new GP will be needed when entering residential care, however.

Preparation also includes psychological adjustment to the placement process. For many carers, placement is seen as an admission of failure; they feel that they have let the dementing person down, that they are selfish, that they are abandoning their loved one. These emotions are understandable but in most circumstances are not accurate reflections of what has been happening. Carers may need to work through these emotions with a counsellor to avoid inappropriate self-blame from developing. Other carers are able to see that they have done as much as they can to look after the dementing person at home and are able to focus on the next step. Research shows that most carers adjust to the placement and after about six months are much less stressed than they were beforehand.

The dementing person can often be gradually prepared for the placement by the carer and health professionals talking about the topic from time to time to gauge their receptivity. This may have to be subtle because some people are very sensitive about the issue and may flare up at the mere mention of residential placement. A method that works for some people is to use residential respite as a gradual introduction to permanent placement. For others, an initial placement for temporary respite care may turn into permanent residential care without going home again. In this regard, it is often noted that a dementing person's outright opposition to placement disappears after being in residential care for a week or two, as illustrated in the following case.

Christine lived alone and was supported by her only daughter Kay and a Community Aged Care Package. It was clear to all involved that despite their best efforts, Christine was becoming very unsafe at home. She would be up in the middle of the night and in her anxious confusion would ring Kay repeatedly. During the day she wandered from her home, having to be brought back by the police on several occasions. Although Kay had considered taking her mother to her home, there really wasn't enough room and Christine objected. She was equally vehement in her refusal to consider placement. After months of persuasion, and a fortuitous accident in which she flooded her kitchen, necessitating major repairs, Christine reluctantly agreed to a temporary placement until the kitchen was fixed. She was initially unsettled in the new environment but after a week seemed quite content. Indeed, she commented to Kay 'how nice they all were'. After some weeks, during which time she made no mention of going back home, the respite placement was converted to a permanent placement.

Of course, there are many variants to this scenario. Another common outcome is for the dementing person to remain unhappy about staying but no longer raise objections to it. In other cases, little planning is possible when an unexpected medical complication develops, for example a stroke, and the combination of medical problems and dementia means community care is no longer feasible. Many dementing people are placed into residential care from acute hospitals. One of the reasons for this is that it is generally easier to place a person in an unfamiliar environment when they are recovering from illness. Hospital doctors and nurses may more easily persuade the dementing person at a time when they are feeling less well in themselves and not up to self-care for a while.

REQUIREMENTS OF GOOD RESIDENTIAL CARE

There are two main requirements of good residential care. The first involves the delivery of quality professional health and personal care. The second involves ensuring that the residential care environment is as 'home like' as possible without compromising safety.

Professional health and personal care

The attitudes, knowledge and skills of the staff are probably the most important asset of any aged care facility. The delivery of quality care requires well-trained staff who have a positive attitude towards older people with dementia and respect their rights. These two aspects of personal care—quality care and protection of resident rights—form the basis of residential care standards in Australia.[2]

Facilities vary in the level of professional supervision and personal care they provide. It is important for residents to retain as much autonomy as possible, so the degree of professional involvement varies according to functional need. Some facilities are intended to provide minimal levels of professional involvement for people who are functionally independent with limited supervision, while others are set up to provide high-level care for people fully dependent in their activities of daily living such as bathing, feeding and toileting. Of course, the less professional care required, the less expensive it is to run the facility, so there are financial aspects too whereby the funding source, which in Australia is mainly the Commonwealth Government, is keen to cap its costs. Occasionally some older people have the mistaken impression that they are going to be looked after as if they were in a hotel or private residence, with servants there to respond to their every wish. This often leads to conflicts with the staff, who resent being ordered around, particularly by a person capable of self-care.

There is a gradation of care from low to high level depending on the individual needs of the resident. By the time a resident needs high-level care, health professional involvement, mainly nursing, is required many times during the day. In all levels of care, specific training in dementia management is important, though this can be difficult to achieve as many staff remain for only a few years.

There is a lot of research demonstrating very high stress levels in staff who work in aged care facilities.[3] Morale can become a problem in some facilities and low morale is often linked with suboptimal care. In addition, with the current worldwide nursing shortages, many facilities are short staffed. Pay rates are also relatively low, so recruitment and retention of staff can be a problem. All of this has been exacerbated in Australia by the removal of regulations about nursing levels, which some authorities believe has encouraged understaffing in some facilities as a cost-saving device.

Facility design and atmosphere

For many years, residential care design seemed to have been dictated by staff and administrative considerations rather than by the needs of residents, and so many facilities were sterile and institutional. Thankfully, designs over the last fifteen or so years have improved considerably, with a better balance being achieved between the needs of staff, administrators and residents, though costs often limit what can be done. This has been partially driven by more vigorous government standards for nursing home design, but also by the belated recognition that aged care facilities are the residents' homes.

So, what design features are believed to assist in the care of people with dementia?[4] One of the more important aspects of design is for it to be 'home-like'. The problem is that people come from diverse backgrounds and home conditions, thus there isn't a single design that fits all. This is amplified by our multicultural society, where the cultural traditions of different ethnic groups may be best met either by facilities specifically designed for one

Table 11.1 Dementia-friendly features in aged care facilities

'Home-like'	Consider culture, food, language, religion
'Age-appropriate'	Consider colour scheme, fittings and furnishings
Lighting	Avoid too bright (glare/shadows) or too dark, need dim nightlights
Acoustics	No reverberating sound; avoid public address system
Size	Dementia-specific unit for 6–15 residents
Security	If needed, secure doors, electronic tags
Sight-lines	Able to see most important sections (bedroom, dining room, toilet) from living area; avoid long corridors, many corners, recessed doors
Floors	Non-slippery, no distracting patterns, no little steps
Toilets/bathrooms	Good signage, wheelchair access, grab bars
Living rooms	More than one needed; different-sized comfortable chairs (not too low), TV, radio, video
Dining areas	Allow both communal and individual meals
Outside space	Gardens, paths, seats, security
Activities	Check the social and activity program, community and carer involvement
Staff	Ask about training program; note involvement of staff with residents and staff attitudes

group, or by sections of a facility being set aside for a particular group. Other reasons for needing culture-specific facilities include language, food, religion and other traditions.

Another design feature touted for dementia is 'age-appropriateness', whereby the facility is intended to remind the dementing person of their younger adult days through the colour schemes, fittings and furnishings, on the presumption that this will put them more at ease. The dilemma here is that there may be a 30-year age spread among residents in the one facility, so its design might have to incorporate the era from the 1920s to the 1950s, a period in which many home changes occurred. A person who might feel quite at ease with typical designs of the 1920s might be irritated by 1950s designs. This is likely to become a bigger issue in the future, as design changes accelerated in the 1960s and 1970s. I shudder to think what might transpire if the psychedelic patterns of this era were re-created—though it may well be that people who lived through that era are more used to dealing with change and will be able to cope with it.

Designs need to compensate for the cognitive deficits and challenging behaviour of dementia while allowing staff to have good visual access. Lighting should be sufficient to avoid dark areas, but not too bright, which can lead to problems with glare and shadows. Dim nightlights might minimise nocturnal confusion. Poor acoustics are a problem, especially where you have uncontrolled noise from residents in the severe stage of dementia who scream. The use of public address systems for staff communication can add to the problem, so wall and ceiling materials that absorb sound are important.

The number of persons to be housed in an area is very important. The ideal size of a facility primarily intended for persons with challenging behaviour is from six to fifteen residents. This usually means that it is a self-contained part of a larger facility. If the facility is required for a person who wanders, the doors need to be locked with either a combination lock, security swipe card or keyed access. When challenging behaviour is not an issue, 20 to 25 residents can be reasonably looked after in one section. The overall design should be kept as simple as possible—complexes with long corridors with many corners and recessed doors are hard enough for the staff to find their way around, let alone the residents! Walking surfaces need to be even and without distracting patterns or a tendency to produce glare. Small steps that are difficult to see may be unsafe.

Toilets should be easily accessible, with good signage, and preferably visible from bedrooms, activity and living areas so that residents have a better chance of avoiding 'accidents'. Bathrooms need standard safety features including grab bars, non-slip tubs and showers with wheelchair access.

There must be quiet areas of various sizes for residents to sit comfortably in varying degrees of privacy. The seating itself should be safe and comfortable. While recliner chairs may have an important role with dementing people who are unable to ambulate, they can be dangerous, as they are difficult to get out of and falls may occur. Dining areas should allow for both communal and individual meals, as some people are more comfortable eating in company and others alone.

Secure outside space, preferably with well-designed gardens, rest spots and walking paths, is important for exercise and to assist with some challenging behaviour such as restlessness. Flower and herb gardens also provide excellent sensory stimulation. Other features that can make a facility more home-like include pets, indoor plants, encouraging residents to help with chores, and policies that encourage open interaction with the local community, including visits from schoolchildren, volunteer groups and church groups.

Another factor that impinges upon facility design is the concept of 'ageing in place', which refers to the dementing person remaining in the one facility until they die. This can be most successfully achieved in a larger facility with sections for low-level and high-level care. Some dementia facilities, particularly those that cater for challenging behaviours, do not provide care for persons who are bedbound with advanced dementia, and require the person to be transferred to another facility.

The downside of creating a home-like atmosphere is that such a design may increase the risk of accidents by incorporating furniture and fittings that are easy to trip over. Falls resulting in hip fractures are a major problem in nursing homes. Although hip surgery has improved considerably, it is sobering to realise that about one-third of older people with hip fractures die within twelve months.

Certain features, such as pets, may not appeal to all residents and there is always the fear that atypical infections such as scabies might be acquired from a pet. Another problem is that tough (some might say pedantic) regulations may prevent particular resident activities. Meredith Gresham, an occupational therapist, told me of an experience in a residential facility in the United States where she encouraged some residents to assist in meal preparation—only to be told that State legislation forbade the residents from eating the food due to hygiene concerns! Obviously there needs to be a balance between creating a safe, hygienic environment backed up by appropriate regulations and the provision of optimal quality of life through a home-like atmosphere.

TYPES OF RESIDENTIAL CARE FOR DEMENTIA

The type of facility that is appropriate for an individual will vary depending upon the severity of the dementia and the degree of behavioural complications. Facilities designed for wanderers need to be secure, with ample space for them to exercise safely both indoors and outdoors. On the other hand, a person with severe dementia who doesn't wander, or has limited mobility and no other major challenging behaviour, can often be managed in a mainstream facility. Indeed, most if not all aged care facilities in Australia have a large proportion of residents with dementia. Hence, all facilities need to have design features to assist in dementia care, though such features are extremely variable from one facility to the next. While many aged care facilities specialise in either high-level or low-level care, some cover both. The latter was encouraged by the 1997 *Aged Care Act*, which was designed to better integrate the hostel (low-level care) and nursing home (high-level care) sectors.[5]

Low-level care aged care facilities

These facilities (formerly known as hostels) are not specifically intended for persons with dementia but in reality about 28 per cent of residents have dementia.[6] Thus a well-designed low-level care facility should have many of the features previously described for dementia. Some will even have locked doors, though this tends to impinge upon the rights of residents who are not demented.

Individual residents have their own rooms with en suite bathrooms. Most are designed like bed-sitters with a section of the room used as a living area and the rest as a bedroom. Sometimes there is a kitchenette. The size varies between facilities and in some of the older ones the rooms can be quite small. Indeed, a number of facilities around Australia have had to undertake major refurbishments to meet new Commonwealth accreditation guidelines. Residents are usually encouraged to use their own furniture from home to assist in the settling-in process, particularly items such as TVs, stereos, sideboards, bookcases, coffee tables, lounge chairs, pictures and mementos. Obviously not much can fit into one room so difficult choices often have to be made.

Professional supervision may be largely limited to medication administration. There is minimal health professional involvement from day to day. Personal care assistants might ensure that the residents have their meals, are looking after their personal hygiene and are participating in social activities organised by the facility. Assistance with specific aspects of personal care will be given if required. As many dementing residents have some challenging behaviour, there is often a need for the staff to have a plan of behaviour management.

In my experience, most physically fit people with mild–moderate dementia who require residential care rather than living alone are well suited to this type of care. Another group this type of care might suit is married couples, when the carer is too frail to continue care at home. Often adjoining or shared rooms can be arranged.

High-level care aged care facilities

At least 60 per cent of residents in these facilities (formerly known as nursing homes) have dementia.[7] Many others have milder mental impairments due to stroke, Parkinson's disease and other medical conditions. It is important to realise that most people with dementia do not require dementia-specific facilities, as described below. Unless there are particular behavioural concerns that require specific care, standard high-level aged care facilities are equipped to manage them.

The main difference between low-level and high-level care is the amount of assistance required for the resident. In general, most persons with severe dementia and many with moderate dementia require high-level care, needing assistance with eating, dressing, bathing, toileting and often mobility. Many residents are chairbound or bedbound and require two people to move them, often with the aid of a mechanical lifter. While personal care and nursing assistants can accomplish many of these tasks, there is also a need for registered nurses to be present full-time to manage medications, change catheters, apply dressings, administer special feeds and provide overall supervision of the other staff. This will involve regular interactions with the residents' GPs and medical specialists as well as with their families and friends. Other health professionals required in high-level facilities include physiotherapists (particularly to assist with rehabilitation), diversional therapists and music therapists.

Dementia-specific facilities

Dementia-specific facilities include special care units, psychogeriatric aged care facilities, Confused and Disturbed Elderly

(CADE) Units and psychogeriatric extended care units, all of which cater for dementing persons with behavioural disturbances too severe to be managed in standard aged care facilities. Such behaviours included severe aggression, marked agitation and incessant wandering. About 6 per cent of high-level care facilities are dementia-specific; so also are about 5 per cent of low-level care facilities, for apart from the behavioural disturbance the dementing person may still be relatively independent.[8] Some people are of the opinion that any person with a dementia diagnosis should be in this type of facility. This is unnecessary, as there is no evidence that such units are any better than a standard aged care facility for the average person with dementia.[9] As described earlier, dementia-specific units should be small (catering for between six and fifteen residents) and self-contained, although usually part of a larger facility. Units of larger size are likely to amplify the behaviours they are intended to deal with. The staff needs to have specific training and expertise in the management of behavioural disturbances. In addition, staff numbers have to be higher than average to ensure that the individual residents get sufficient attention in a safe manner.

In my opinion, dementia-specific facilities should not be viewed as permanent placement. Most severe behavioural disturbances subside with a combination of good management and time, and after six to twelve months most residents have improved sufficiently to be managed in a standard facility. Unfortunately, this doesn't tend to happen, and most dementia-specific facilities, particularly those in the private sector, have many residents who no longer need to be there—or indeed didn't really need to be there in the first place. This tends to block access for the persons who really need them, who are then often inappropriately placed in standard facilities where major problems ensue. In some states, such as Victoria, local Aged Care Mental Health Services are involved in managing these facilities and act as gatekeepers. This allows more appropriate use of the resource for the broader community and it is the process favoured by most professional advocates.

THE RESIDENTIAL CARE SYSTEM IN AUSTRALIA

All admissions to residential care require an Aged Care Client Record to be completed by an ACAT that indicates whether the approval is for high-level or low-level care. This forms the basis of Commonwealth funding to the aged care facility, with residents assessed as low-level care being funded at this level. The precise level of funding an aged care facility receives from the Commonwealth is based upon a complex assessment process using a tool called the Resident Classification Scale (RCS), applied by the aged care facility staff over the first 21 days of admission. The RCS covers issues such as communication, continence, mobility, feeding, social needs and behaviour and requires detailed daily documentation from the nursing staff on each of its 20 items. From this, eight categories of care for funding are defined, with Classification Levels 1–4 being high level and Classification Levels 5–8 being low level. These classifications remain valid for twelve months, at which time the process is repeated. Residents initially assessed as requiring low-level care by an ACAT but later found to be requiring high-level care can be reassessed by the ACAT.[10]

The documentation required is so time consuming that it has been roundly criticised by coalface staff for taking them away from the residents they are supposed to be looking after. Another criticism is that despite a revision a few years ago, the RCS is still regarded as not giving sufficient funding for the management of behavioural problems. Fortunately, in May 2002 the Federal Minister for Ageing, Kevin Andrews, announced that the Department of Health and Ageing would set up a review of the RCS to examine ways of relieving the paperwork burden. It is intended that new options will be piloted in 2003.[11]

RESIDENT FEES AND CHARGES

There are three components to the fees and charges that may be levied from residents of aged care facilities—the basic daily care fee, the daily income-tested fee, and accommodation payments. These vary according to the income and assets of the resident.[12]

Basic daily care fee

This is a contribution to the cost of care. At 20 March 2003, the means-tested pensioner fee was a maximum of $25.73 per day and the non-pensioner fee was a maximum of $32.12 per day.

Daily income-tested fee

This is another contribution to the cost of care but is paid only by part-pensioners and non-pensioners. At 20 March 2003, the part-pensioner fee was a maximum of $19.91 per day, with the maximum fee being payable by single part-pensioners with income from $32 005 per annum and married part-pensioners with combined income from $63 282 per annum. The non-pensioner fee was a maximum of $45.07 per day, with the maximum fee being payable by single non-pensioners with income of $68 638 per annum and married non-pensioners with combined income of $136 548 per annum.

Resident accommodation payments

Accommodation payments are also obtained from residents as a contribution towards the cost of their care. Before 1997, there were no accommodation payments in high-level care though they had been in place in low-level care for some time. At the time, the decision to introduce accommodation charges in high-level care was controversial but necessary to assist in improving the capital funding streams to upgrade and replace nursing homes that were rapidly decaying. It also removed the inequity between low-level and high-level care payments.

There are two types of means-tested accommodation payments: accommodation bonds and accommodation charges.

Accommodation bonds

These are for people who permanently enter low-level care or enter an extra-services home, which is a facility that is able to charge residents higher fees for extra 'hotel' type services. Accommodation bonds are akin to an interest-free loan given to the aged care facility, provided that the facility meets minimum building and care standards. The residential care service provider may keep up to $246 a month from the bond for up to five years, known as the retention period. When the resident leaves the home, the remainder is refunded.

There is no set amount for an accommodation bond, but its payment cannot leave the resident with less than $27 500 in assets.

This includes the resident's home, unless: the resident's spouse or dependent child is living in the private home; a carer eligible for an income support payment has lived there for two years; or a close relative who is eligible for an income support payment has been living there for at least five years. In these situations, the resident's home is excluded as an asset. Persons with less than $27 500 in assets are called concessional residents and do not pay the bond. Each aged care facility must take a minimum number of concessional residents, for whom they obtain additional Commonwealth subsidy.

Residents must enter a bond agreement, which sets out their rights and responsibilities, within seven days of entering the facility. The bonds can be paid as lump sums, fortnightly payments or a combination of the two. Residents have up to six months to pay the bond as a lump sum, though interest may be charged. If the resident transfers to another low-level aged care facility, the bond is transferred and the resident cannot be asked to pay a higher amount. If the resident moves to high-level care, either the bond can be transferred as described before or the balance fully refunded and the resident can pay the daily accommodation charge in the new aged care home for a period of up to five years.

Aged care facilities must have prudential arrangements in place and guarantee in writing to repay the bond balance within statutory time periods, which are within seven days if a resident transfers to another home or two months in any other circumstances.

Accommodation charges

These are paid for up to five years by residents entering high-level care, providing the aged care facility meets minimum building and care standards. There is a means test similar to that applied to the accommodation bond, and residents with less than $27 500 in assets do not have to pay the accommodation charge. Others who don't have to pay include residents who were in a nursing home prior to 30 September 1997, and those paying the accommodation bond in an extra-services home. The maximum accommodation charge payable at 20 March 2003 was $13.45 per day (about $4900 per year) and applies to residents with assets of $52 046 or more. Assisted residents, who are means-tested pensioners who have not owned their own home in the previous two years and have assets between $27 500 and $44 000, are charged on a sliding scale up to a maximum of $6.73 per day. For married residents, half the couple's combined assets are counted, though the family home is excluded if the partner or dependent child is still living there. The family home is also excluded for carers and other relatives as described previously under the accommodation bond.

Payment of accommodation charges can be deferred and paid out of the resident's estate. In these circumstances, the aged care facility is entitled to charge interest at no more than double the lowest pension deeming rate, as determined by the Commonwealth Government, applicable at the time of entering the facility.

One important issue with accommodation bonds and charges is that the dementing person needs to have sufficient mental competence to sign the agreement with the aged care facility. If the dementing person is mentally incompetent, a guardian or enduring power of attorney will need to sign the agreement on their behalf.

QUALITY IN AGED CARE FACILITIES

This has been a controversial area in recent years, with a series of incidents of poor quality care in aged care facilities being highlighted in the media. Stringent regulations provide minimum standards for the provision of care and accommodation in aged care facilities, but it seems that their monitoring and enforcement has not always been optimal.

Accommodation

All aged care facilities have to be certified by inspection to meet minimum building standards related to fire safety, security, resident privacy, occupational health and safety, lighting, heating, cooling and ventilation. In 1998, a ten-year plan was announced to improve the privacy and space requirements for residents. While most low-level care facilities already meet the requirements, high-level care facilities are in general much older stock, with over 90 per cent of them more than ten years old. Thus in 1997, while 97 per cent of low-level care residents were in single rooms, only 24 per cent of high-level care residents had the same privilege and over 33 per cent were in rooms with three or more residents, with the proposed maximum to be achieved by 2008 being two per room. A new certification instrument was introduced in July 1999 with a pass mark of 60 per cent, including a mandatory fire safety minimum score of 78 per cent. By the end of 2003, all aged care facilities will have been inspected with this instrument. There is already good evidence that significant improvements are occurring in both the standard of new facilities and the refurbishment of old. The capital made available by accommodation bonds and charges appears to be having the desired effect on building upgrades.[13]

Accreditation and quality of care

Since 1997, accreditation of aged care facilities has been based on the philosophy of continuous improvement. Quality care is defined as being provided when the standards of care specified in the 1997 *Aged Care Act* legislation are met. These are outcome standards that embrace management systems, staffing, organisational development, health, personal care and lifestyle of residents, the physical environment and safety systems. The Aged Care Standards and Accreditation Agency is a body independent of government and the residential aged care industry, and was set up to manage the accreditation process. Aged care facilities are accredited for periods of one to three years depending on how well they are assessed to be performing. Where inadequate care is identified, this is publicised and made available on the Department of Health and Aged Care website (see Appendix 1). Sanctions can be imposed; for example, an aged care facility which does not meet the standards may be prevented from admitting new residents until certain improvements are made. There is always the option of closing the facility if conditions warrant it, as occurred in one Victorian facility, but this might impose greater hardship on the residents as they have to be found alternative care. On the other side of the coin, where commendations for good care are made these are also publicised. As with the collection of information for the RCS, the bureaucratic demands of the accreditation process seem to outweigh some of its usefulness by distracting the staff from resident care and by increasing costs (the aged care facilities have to pay to be accredited).[14]

FUTURE CONCERNS

There are a number of concerns regarding the future of residential aged care in Australia.[15]

- In the 1980s there was clearly an oversupply of high-level aged care facilities and consequently there was a clamping down on the number of bed licences granted, a situation that continues to this day. Now there is an emerging undersupply of beds with consequent pressures on carers and acute hospitals being blocked up with people awaiting a place.
- Despite improvements in funding of high-level aged care facilities through the accommodation payments, there are still major concerns that there is inadequate investment, both governmental and non-governmental, in the industry. Much more capital investment is required for building improvements.
- Although nursing shortages are worldwide, the residential aged care sector has greater problems in attracting and retaining staff due to the nature of the work and the relatively poor (compared to acute hospitals) pay rates. The high staff turnover endemic in many facilities further exacerbates the difficulties in implementing effective training programs essential to improving dementia care.

SUMMARY

For many reasons it is a good idea for carers to prepare for residential care well before it is needed. This should involve finding out about local facilities and becoming informed about facility features indicative of quality care. There are generally three types of residential aged care facilities in Australia—low-level (hostel), high-level (nursing home) and dementia-specific facilities. Only residents with severe behavioural problems need the latter. All admissions to aged care facilities have to be assessed by an Aged Care Assessment Team beforehand to determine the level of care required. Residential aged care in Australia is subsidised by the Commonwealth with means-tested fees and charges for the accommodation and care for the resident. An accreditation process monitors the quality of care.

CHAPTER 12

ETHICAL AND LEGAL ISSUES

ETHICAL PRINCIPLES

A number of ethical principles underpin the way we lead our lives. One of the most important of these is *autonomy*, which is the individual's right to be self-governing, in other words to exercise self-direction, freedom and moral independence. Because dementia fundamentally impairs the capacity of an individual to be autonomous, many ethical and legal problems that arise in dementia care occur around this principle due to conflicts involving decision-making capacity. For example, competency to manage finances, to drive a car, to participate in research and to decide where to live are common areas of concern, discussed later in this chapter.

Other ethical principles that have direct bearing on many of these situations also need to be considered. For carers and health professionals, *beneficence*, which means doing good or conferring benefits that enhance personal or social well-being, and *non-maleficence*, which means doing no harm, are often the ethical basis of the care being provided. Sometimes these principles may come into conflict and at these times the principle of *justice* may come into play. Justice is about fairness and impartiality and the need to find a balance between competing interests; examples include balancing the desire of the dementing person to live alone in their own home with the concerns of carers about hygiene and safety, and balancing the potential benefits of a drug treatment against the risk of serious side-effects. Ultimately, when a dementing person is found to be incompetent to make a particular decision, it is essential that the needs of the dementing person, rather than the needs of carers, health professionals or others, be the basis for the decision that is arrived at—in other words, the decision must provide a just outcome for the dementing person.[1]

MENTAL COMPETENCY: DECISION-MAKING CAPACITY

A fundamental impact of dementia upon an individual is to impair their decision-making capacity and hence their ability to remain autonomous. To have the mental capacity to make a decision, the person must be capable of understanding the nature of the decision and the effects that the decision will have upon themselves and others.[3] It is important to understand that mental competence is not 'all or nothing'. For example, a dementing person may be mentally incompetent to make a will but competent to decide whether to give their power of attorney to their spouse. It is crucial in respecting the autonomy of the dementing person to ensure that they retain their rights to make decisions about things they remain competent to decide upon. A dementing person whose finances are managed by a guardian, for example, may be able to decide where they want to live or what medical treatment they wish to receive. The guardian in these circumstances should not attempt to impose their will upon the dementing person, although of course they have the right to provide their views on the matter.

HOW IS DECISION-MAKING CAPACITY DETERMINED?

Peteris Darzins from the National Ageing Research Institute in Melbourne and colleagues from Canada have provided lucid practical guidelines for the assessment of mental capacity with 'The 6-Step Capacity Assessment Process'.[3] These guidelines are easy to follow, sensible and fair. Although competency assessments can be made by a variety of health professionals, medical specialists, in particular psychiatrists, usually perform them. It is useful for family carers to understand the process as well.

Step 1: Is there a trigger to make an assessment?

I have often been asked by family carers to assess whether their relative is competent to make a will at a time when the relative has no plans to make a will. In these circumstances I suggest they return when there is a plan to make a will, as an assessment is otherwise of little value. In other words, there needs to be a valid trigger for the assessment. There is no need to make any competency assessment without such a trigger. Valid triggers may include concerns about the person's ability to make financial decisions after bills have been left unpaid, or concerns about the dementing person's apparent inability to make appropriate critical decisions about personal care.

Step 2: Engage the dementing person in the process

This means that the dementing person should be adequately informed about the reason for the assessment and efforts made to gain their assent to participate in the process. This step needs to be handled with some delicacy, as many individuals will become indignant and defensive when their competency is questioned. Sometimes carers wish to avoid this step on the grounds that the person's mental incompetence is self-evident and they do not want to upset them by the examination. While the sentiments are understandable, this approach would deny the dementing person the right to be properly assessed.

Step 3: Information gathering

To determine competency, the assessor needs as much information as possible about the situation. This is particularly important with assessments for the capacity to make a will (testamentary capacity), where full knowledge of the person's assets and their natural beneficiaries is needed. However, it is not only information of a factual nature that is required, but also the attitudes, values and goals of the person being assessed. In this area, carers can provide valuable information.

Step 4: Education

The importance of this step is that the dementing person is given every opportunity to demonstrate their competence by being provided with adequate information about the situation. Sometimes dementing people appear to be making incompetent decisions but when fully informed of the ramifications of the decision they were apparently going to make, change their mind to a decision that is competent. Ignorance should not be allowed to be the basis of a competency decision. Often carers are not aware that lack of knowledge lies behind what appears to be a stubborn refusal to 'do the right thing'. Nor should reasonable indecision about which medical treatment to follow be the basis of a competency decision. A diagnosis of cancer can lead to prolonged indecision about treatment in fully competent people so it should not be surprising that a person with dementia might have similar difficulty.

Step 5: Capacity assessment

In this step, the assessor tests the dementing person's ability to make the decision by seeing how well they understand or appreciate the decisions they face. If the dementing person does not understand the ramifications of their decision, nor appreciate the effects the decision will have upon others, then they are incompetent to make that particular decision.

Step 6: Acting on the results of the capacity assessment

The results of the assessment may confirm the dementing person's competence to make the decision and this should be conveyed to those who expressed the initial concern. If the dementing person is found to be incompetent, the capacity assessment will form the basis of the appointment of a substitute decision maker. Importantly, even if the dementing person is incompetent to make a particular decision, they may have views about the issue that need to be taken into account by the appointed substitute decision maker. For example, the dementing person may not be competent to decide whether they should be in a nursing home, but may be able to indicate that they would prefer to live in a certain locality.

SUBSTITUTE DECISION MAKERS

In Australia, each State and Territory jurisdiction has its own legislation providing the legal basis for the appointment of a substitute decision maker; while there are some differences around the country the general approach is similar. Thus I explain some of the common terms used in this area and list contact points in Appendices 1 and 2.

Is it essential that a substitute decision maker be appointed? In many circumstances decisions for dementing persons are made by informal carers without any legal appointment but with the obvious blessing of the dementing person. Often it is the spouse in this situation and, providing the couple have joint bank accounts to enable the spouse to access finances and the dementing person does not overtly object to any decisions made by the spouse, this may suffice. In some jurisdictions this informal decision making is recognised in legislation. In New South Wales, the *Guardianship Act* describes such decision makers for medical and dental treatment as the 'person responsible' (as opposed to 'next of kin', which fails to recognise that at times the person in the best position to make a decision will not be a relative) and provides a hierarchy for determining who this should be. At the top of the hierarchy is the spouse or de facto spouse, providing there is a close and continuing relationship with the person. Next on the hierarchy is the carer or person who arranges care on a regular basis and is unpaid (not including carer's payments), or arranged such care before the person was admitted to residential care; and finally a close friend or relative.[4] However, particularly for financial management, it is highly recommended that formal legal arrangements are made as described below.

ADVANCE HEALTH CARE DIRECTIVES

Sometimes called a 'living will', an advanced health care directive is a written statement made by a competent person about what medical treatment they would like to receive when they are no longer competent to make the decision. For a dementing person, it would be wise to cover end-of-life issues such as resuscitation, tube feeding and intravenous therapy. These directives are not backed by legislation in all States of Australia, but when medical decisions are made for an incompetent person, the views expressed, written when the person was competent, should always be taken into account by the substitute decision maker. If a competent person wishes to make an advance directive, it is advisable to gain medical and legal advice about the format.[5]

POWER OF ATTORNEY AND ENDURING POWER OF ATTORNEY

A power of attorney is a legal document by which a mentally competent person authorises someone to make financial decisions and sign papers on their behalf. However, a power of attorney becomes invalid if a dementing person loses their decision-making capacity. For this reason, people with dementia need to authorise an enduring power of attorney, a document that contains a statement that the authorisation will continue when they lose their mental capacity. An enduring power of attorney needs to be completed with a 'prescribed person', usually a solicitor, barrister or clerk of the Local Court. In some States, such as New South Wales, an enduring power of attorney applies only to financial decision making; in other States, such as Western Australia, it is equivalent to an enduring guardianship. The enduring power of attorney may need to be registered if land deals are to be transacted with it. As with advance directives and enduring guardianship, an enduring power of attorney may be revoked while the person remains competent.[6]

The person entrusted with enduring power of attorney is usually a family member or close friend. Where an older person has no one to turn to, or does not wish to encumber family or friends, there are several options available, including the dementing person's solicitor or accountant or the Public Trustee, to act as the enduring power of attorney and look after their financial affairs.

ENDURING GUARDIANSHIP

In some States of Australia a mentally competent person may appoint someone known as an enduring guardian (in other States known as enduring power of attorney) to make personal, lifestyle and medical treatment decisions when they are no longer able to make these decisions themselves. While this assures the dementing person about the identity of the person who will make the decisions, it does not specifically guarantee the content of the decisions, though some written directives might help guide the decision making (such as with an advance health care directive) and the conditions or limitations the person desires. In New South Wales, for example, enduring guardianship must be in writing, in an approved form, with a legal witness. Enduring guardianship only comes into effect when the person loses their competence; until that time the dementing person may change their mind and revoke it in writing with a legal witness.[7]

GUARDIANSHIP

When a person with dementia no longer has the capacity to make a decision and no formal arrangements are in place for a substitute decision maker (for example, an enduring power of attorney), in most circumstances their informal carer, usually a spouse or child, is able to make many decisions on their behalf. However, when the dementing person objects to the lifestyle decision being made, or when financial transactions have to be undertaken using their resources, a legally appointed guardian is required.

Guardianship legislation varies from State to State but there are many features in common.[8] Usually there are two components—financial management, and personal, lifestyle and medical treatment decisions. In many cases, it is only financial decisions that require the appointment of a legal guardian, for example, when a house must be sold to enable nursing home placement. In this situation a guardian would be appointed with powers limited to this area. At other times guardianship will include lifestyle decisions, for example medical consent. Two types of guardian can be appointed—a family member/friend of the dementing person or a public guardian. Public guardians are usually only appointed in the absence of family/friends or where there is a serious and unresolvable dispute between family/friends about the dementing person. This latter situation includes cases where there has been elder abuse.

The guardianship process can be lengthy, though urgent hearings can be obtained in an emergency, at which an interim guardian may be appointed until the situation is fully investigated—for example, where it is suspected that a dementing person is being defrauded. There are two basic criteria to be met. First, it is necessary to establish that the dementing person is unable to make a competent decision due to the effects of their illness. This usually requires two health professional reports to establish the extent of the disability. Second, it is necessary to demonstrate a need to appoint a guardian, that is, that there are decisions to be made which an informal carer is legally unable to make. Information is gathered about the situation and a tribunal hearing is held which all interested parties, including the dementing person, are encouraged to attend. The tribunal usually includes a lawyer, a health professional and a lay person on the panel. If the tribunal determines that a guardian should be appointed, it then determines who should be the appointed guardian and the extent of the guardian's powers. For example, if it is intended that the guardian have the power to authorise nursing home placement against the dementing person's will, this must usually be explicitly stated in the guardianship order. If a decision required lies outside the guardian's appointed powers, this will have to be considered by the tribunal.

DRIVING

There is no doubt that dementia adversely affects a person's ability to drive. The unresolved question is at what point the dementing person should cease to drive. The American Academy of Neurology has recommended that all persons diagnosed with dementia should cease driving; in the State of California, the diagnosing doctor must report a diagnosis of Alzheimer's disease, which usually results in revocation of the driving licence.[9] Given that many people are being diagnosed with very mild dementia these days, mandatory licence revocation appears harsh, as many of them would still be capable of driving safely.

In Australia, the medical standards for cognitive impairment and dementia recommend that 'patients should not drive if there is significant impairment of memory, visuospatial skills, insight or judgement or if there are problematic hallucinations or delusions'. It is also stated that baseline and regular review are required. If there are any doubts, a driving assessment is suggested. If the dementing person refuses a driving assessment, 'consideration should be given to reporting the matter to the driver licensing authority'.[10] Thus there is no obligatory reporting and the standards allow considerable leeway to medical practitioners. However, a medical practitioner may be liable under civil law in cases where a court forms the opinion that reasonable steps have not been taken to stop an impaired person from driving.

There are numerous potential consequences to having driving privileges revoked.[11] Loss of independence is the major problem.

It may be difficult to find alternative transport, though for many people it may well be cheaper to use taxis than to maintain a car. Taxis may be fine for city dwellers, but in rural settings they are not usually a viable option. There are still many older women who have never obtained their driver's licence; when their spouse is no longer able to drive they can become isolated as well. It is not uncommon in such cases to be asked to allow the dementing person to keep driving providing the spouse always travels with them. Loss of the licence can put stress on other family members who may find themselves providing alternative transport. Driving has long been a symbol of independence, particularly for men: loss of the right to drive can be shattering, particularly in an otherwise fit person. Some people become quite depressed, as it often symbolises the decline in function that has been occurring in other ways.

Joe was a 65-year-old retired motor mechanic who had been diagnosed with Alzheimer's disease for a year. Cars had been his life. He fixed them, drove them, watched the Formula 1 Grand Prix on television and regularly went to the races at Bathurst. He was proud of his perfect driving record. Joe's wife Dianne had noticed that over the previous six months he seemed less sure of himself while driving. There was nothing too dramatic, just some hesitancy at intersections, uncertainty with new road signs and disorientation in unfamiliar areas. Dianne was usually with him so she was able to help. The situation came to a head when some unexpected roadworks required a detour onto one lane of the other side of the road. Joe was slow to react and, after almost collecting the detour sign, he overcorrected onto the other side of the road, narrowly missing the oncoming traffic. Joe seemed unaware of the extent of his near miss but Dianne realised that there was a problem. After seeking advice, she arranged for Joe to have a driving assessment with an occupational therapist at the regional driving assessment centre. Joe was livid that anyone should doubt his ability to drive but agreed to have the test, during which it became clear that he was repeatedly making errors in complex situations. Even he began to see that he was not driving to his former capacity. Although extremely disappointed when told that he had failed, he accepted the decision and handed in his licence. For months afterwards he was miserable and pining to drive.

The research on the effects of dementia upon driving ability has been inconclusive in many ways. One study conducted in 1997 at Washington University in St Louis, Missouri, demonstrated that while poor driving performance increases with increased severity of dementia, not all people with dementia were unsafe drivers at a given point in time. A second study found that actual crashes do not necessarily occur more frequently in drivers with dementia compared to non-demented elderly drivers, suggesting that the diagnosis of dementia should not be the only reason for revocation of the driving licence. Indeed, it can be difficult to isolate the effects of dementia from other age-related conditions such as poor eyesight and hearing, arthritis, stroke, cardiorespiratory disorders and medication effects. People over the age of 70 have higher rates of road traffic accidents than younger people per kilometre travelled. However, there is evidence that persons with very mild dementia can have problems in on-road tests in dealing with the complexity of unexpected events and multiple road signs. Perception of signs when driving at speed can also be poor.[12]

Unfortunately, simple cognitive tests do not reliably discriminate between safe and unsafe drivers.[13] Some authorities have claimed that tests of attention, visual memory and visuospatial function might identify unsafe drivers, but this has not been confirmed in large studies. Consequently, the only reliable way to tell whether a person with early dementia is safe to drive is by the use of an in-car, on-the-road evaluation or other functional test to assess driving skills. One of the dilemmas here is that there seems to be great variability in driving assessments, depending on such factors as the jurisdiction in which they occur and whether they are performed by occupational therapists who specialise in assessing dementing people or by regular driving assessors from the licensing authority who, it seems, can be extremely lenient in their assessments. This is an area that requires better standards.

It should be remembered that driving is a privilege, not a right. Individuals who have chronic progressive disorders such as dementia are obliged to notify the licensing authority of their condition when they believe it impairs their ability to drive safely.[14] Of course, with a condition such as dementia, self-reporting is a rare occurrence.

I believe that all drivers diagnosed with dementia who want to keep driving should undergo a baseline driving assessment in their own car by a driving assessor with expertise in this area, usually an occupational therapist. This should be reviewed annually or earlier if evidence of impaired driving skills emerges through the onset of repeated minor scrapes, for example, or the concerns of an observer. Some people decide of their own accord to stop driving soon after diagnosis. Everyone should be given the opportunity to make up their own mind, providing they are still safe on the road. Raising the issue of driving soon after diagnosis enables such a decision to be made with less stress to all.

Sometimes, no matter how much preparation or planning takes place, the dementing person refuses to accept that they shouldn't drive, even after failing a driving assessment. Various strategies have been used by carers to try to get the message across, including disabling the car, arranging for it to be 'stolen' or sold, getting the local police or some other respected authority figure to speak to the dementing person, and arranging insurance documentation that states the driver is uninsured. Many creative methods have been used; eventually one of them usually works.

RESEARCH ON SUBJECTS WITH DEMENTIA

One of the tenets of medical research, as espoused in various codes of ethics including the World Medical Assembly's Declaration of Helsinki and regulations such as those of Australia's National Health and Medical Research Council, is that participants in such research should give their informed consent. Some people with mild dementia, many with moderate dementia and almost all with severe dementia will have lost the capacity to give their informed consent to participate in research.[15] Most research studies involving new drug treatments for Alzheimer's disease insist that the dementing person be competent to provide informed consent and that the primary carer should provide consent as well. Some worries have been expressed that some participants may lose their decision-making capacity during the course of a long (often six to twelve months) study.[16] Others raise concerns that many participants who appear on the surface to be competent to decide, when examined in greater depth have a very questionable grasp of what is expected of them in the research project. For example, the person with early dementia keen to participate in a trial of a new Alzheimer drug may understand that there is a 50/50 chance of being given an inactive placebo, but may not fully understand the possible side-effects of the new drug, or that alternative treatments are available that do not involve a 50/50 chance of an inactive treatment. It should also be remembered that some new treatments prove to be unsafe when tested in humans, as was discovered in the 'Alzheimer vaccine' trial described in Chapter 2 which resulted in several deaths. In general, however, the approach to drug trials for dementia drugs is seen by most commentators as being ethically sound.

But there are circumstances where the nature of the treatment being studied almost inevitably involves the recruitment of participants incapable of providing informed consent, for example, persons with severe dementia complicated by behavioural disturbances. Is the proxy consent of the spouse or guardian an adequate alternative? Possibly, but while this consent is adequate for accepted treatments, most guardianship legislation does not allow for research consent. The guardianship tribunal in New South Wales is able to make a general decision about whether a specific research study is reasonable to be undertaken in the proposed subjects, leaving it up to the individual's substitute decision maker to give the actual proxy consent. In this situation it is important that the substitute decision maker acts in the dementing person's best interests and not in those of any other party. It has been proposed that advance health care directives should include a clause about a person's willingness or otherwise to participate in research.

Some authorities strongly argue that under no circumstances should persons unable to provide informed consent be allowed to participate in research. The counter-argument runs that this would inevitably mean that very disabled decisionally impaired people would never have the opportunity to benefit from new treatments that have been appropriately researched. In essence, people with severe dementia would be discriminated against.

ELECTRONIC TAGGING

For a long time, many aged care facilities have placed wristbands that contain an electronic tag on dementing people who wander. All the potential exit points of such facilities have boundary alarms that are set off when the tagged person goes through, which allows the staff to bring back the wanderer before they get lost. The advantages of this system are that locked doors and other restraints are avoided. Some concerns have been expressed about loss of liberties but, providing the tags are used judiciously, most authorities believe that this is not an unreasonable approach.[17]

More recently, in the United States electronic tagging has been taken one step further. Silicon chips the size of a grain of rice, which are scanned in much the same way as groceries at a supermarket checkout, are now being implanted into the upper back of dementing people who live in the community. The chips contain identification, contact and medical information in case the person gets lost. Soon the chips will also be capable of being detected by satellite on a global positioning system so the person can be found wherever they are. These developments are a giant leap from the current use of electronic tagging and have much greater ethical concerns related to privacy and autonomy. The potential for misuse seems very high.

PLACEMENT INTO RESIDENTIAL CARE

Few disabled people are keen to leave their own home and move into residential care. Usually it takes a great deal of soul searching on the part of the older person before they can bring themselves to move. Some will stubbornly refuse, even when it is clear to all around that they are living in unsafe circumstances. If the person is mentally competent, however, they have the right to live in whatever way they wish providing it doesn't impinge upon the rights of others.

When a dementing person with impaired decision-making capacity is living alone in an unsafe manner, or with a carer who is very stressed, the dilemma arises as to when placement against their will into residential care is justified. If the dementing person lives alone, carers become understandably concerned about the increased risk of harm through accidents, often much to the chagrin of the dementing person, who resents attempts to impinge on their autonomy. Providing the accident risk doesn't appear to place others at risk of harm, for example, by driving a car, I generally encourage family members to allow risks to be taken in order to respect the person's autonomy.

Ultimately, while community services and carers can ensure

that the home is kept reasonably clean, that food is provided daily, that the laundry is done, bills paid, appointments kept and social activities provided, it is very difficult to prevent accidents occurring during the inevitable long periods that the dementing person is unsupervised. When the risk of harm outweighs the benefits to the person of enjoying their autonomy, it is time to consider placement. Many dementing people who are initially adamantly opposed to placement, if given support and encouragement over some months to consider other options, will eventually change their minds and agree to 'give it a go'. Others will remain stubbornly opposed and, as concerns about safety mount, a guardianship order is usually required to authorise placement. In some States placement might also be achieved under the *Mental Health Act*, with the dementing person being admitted to an acute aged care mental health unit before placement occurs.

When the dementing person is living with a carer, the same principles apply, but the rights of the carer also have to be considered. If the dementing person has a severe behaviour disturbance, for example, exhibiting aggression towards the carer, it is understandable that the carer may get to the point where they are no longer able to tolerate it. Of course, every effort should be made to treat the aggressive behaviour and provide the carer some respite, and in many cases it will be found that the carer has tolerated the behaviour for a long time before seeking help. Where the dementing person would be unable to cope in the absence of the carer, and the carer has come to the end of their tether, it is time for placement.

END-OF-LIFE DECISIONS

Unlike the situation with cancer and other terminal illnesses, planning end-of-life decisions has not often been a routine part of dementia care. This is probably due in part to the difficulty of discussing such issues with a cognitively impaired person and in part to the failure to conceptualise dementia as a terminal illness. Now that early diagnosis is the rule rather than the exception, however, end-of-life decisions can be broached with the dementing person and their family in the form of advanced health care directives as described earlier in the chapter. Nevertheless, many older people are not very comfortable in embracing this approach.

In the absence of an advanced health care directive from the dementing person, a good time for substitute decision makers to discuss end-of-life decisions with medical and nursing staff is at the time of placement into an aged care facility, or possibly during the course of a hospital admission for an intercurrent illness. Issues that should be covered include resuscitation, use of intravenous therapy and tube feeding. In the absence of a 'Do Not Resuscitate' (DNR) order, staff in hospitals in particular but also in aged care facilities are obliged to commence resuscitation; once that process has commenced, it can be difficult to know when to stop. A DNR order prevents unwanted interventions when prolongation of life is not desired.[18]

Most people with severe dementia become impaired in their ability to eat. Weight loss is common but it is not always due to inadequate diet; it seems to be part of the dementing process. Carers become concerned that the dementing person may 'starve to death' and want to do everything possible to prevent that. A swallowing assessment from a speech pathologist is a good initial step to determine the nature of the problem.

Tube feeding is often mentioned as a possible solution. The tube is administered through a technique known as percutaneous endoscopic gastrostomy (PEG), in which a feeding tube is passed through the abdominal wall directly into the stomach. Most authorities believe that tube feeding should not be used to treat dementia-related swallowing difficulties. There is no evidence that tube feeding prevents aspiration of food into the lungs (a common problem in these situations), or increases comfort, weight, quality of life or lifespan. There is evidence that tube feeding results in reduced pleasure from eating, increased use of restraints to prevent the dementing person from removing the tube, and loss of human contact at meal times.

As far as possible, assisted oral feeding is a better approach, though often time consuming. Many family carers visit their relatives daily to feed them; this has the added benefit of providing emotional contact. There comes a time, however, when the dementia is so severe that the dementing person is unable to receive food and water by mouth. It is regarded as ethically permissible to withhold hydration and nutrition in this situation.[19]

Many dementing people die of pneumonia, often related to their immobility, swallowing problems and reduced resistance to infections. Pneumonia can usually be successfully treated with antibiotics and the first or second bout in a nursing home resident is usually treated routinely though often with a perceptible decline in function after each bout. There often comes the point after several bouts of pneumonia when the family, doctor or nurses question whether further antibiotic therapy is warranted. There is no easy answer to this and decisions need to be individually determined by family consultation with the health professionals involved.

SUMMARY

Many ethical and legal problems that arise in dementia care occur around the principle of autonomy due to conflicts involving the decision-making capacity that becomes impaired by the dementia. The appointment of an enduring power of attorney or guardian allied with an advance health care directive during early dementia can avoid many later problems. To have the mental capacity to make a decision, the person must be capable of understanding the nature of the decision and the effects that the decision will have upon themselves and others. A capacity assessment may be required but should only be undertaken with a valid trigger such as concern about financial mismanagement or the need for place-ment into an aged care facility. If the dementing person is found to be incompetent to make the decision, a substitute decision maker should be appointed. Driving assessments should also be undertaken after a dementia diagnosis and repeated at least every year to determine competence to drive. Other ethical issues that commonly occur include end-of-life decisions such as tube feeding.

CHAPTER 13

THE FUTURE

THESE ARE EXCITING TIMES in the field of dementia care. Scarcely a week goes by without the publication of new research findings that provide a better understanding of some aspect of the early diagnosis, potential treatment or prevention of Alzheimer's disease and other dementias. We are on the cusp of being able to reliably identify people *before* they develop symptoms of dementia and, more importantly, being able to provide interventions that will significantly reduce or eliminate their risk of developing dementia. Just how far away this may be and how effective the interventions may be are matters for speculation. In this chapter, with the assistance of some internationally recognised dementia specialists, I provide some educated guesswork about these issues.

DETECTION OF PRE-SYMPTOMATIC INDIVIDUALS AND EARLY DIAGNOSIS

Most experts agree that the accurate detection of individuals with pre-symptomatic dementia is an essential prerequisite for the prevention and successful treatment of various types of dementia, especially Alzheimer's disease. There are a number of ways that this could be achieved, including diagnostic tests of blood, urine or cerebrospinal fluid (CSF); various types of brain scans; and other tests of brain function. It is likely that a combination of approaches might be necessary to achieve sufficient diagnostic accuracy.

These days most people are used to their doctor ordering blood and urine tests that assist in the diagnosis of their medical condition. Some tests are diagnostic of specific illnesses, for example, HIV infection, vitamin B_{12} deficiency, hepatitis-C, though most indicate only a general abnormality that could be due to a range of conditions. In many conditions the precise diagnosis requires a biopsy of the tissue concerned to allow it to be viewed by a pathologist under a microscope. This is usually obtained during a procedure that is designed to be as non-invasive as possible. Most organs of the body are now reasonably accessible for biopsy, either by needle (breast, liver), endoscope, which is a tube introduced through a body orifice (the bowel in a colonoscopy, the stomach in a gastroscopy), or by keyhole surgery (ovaries). Brain biopsies require major surgery, however, and it seems unlikely that any advances in the foreseeable future will allow the safe, reliable biopsy of brain tissue from the desired areas of the brain to allow an accurate diagnosis of dementia during life.

Hence, a considerable amount of research is underway in attempts to find biomarkers for Alzheimer's disease and other dementias. Biomarkers are molecular and biochemical indicators of a disease that can be detected in the blood, urine or CSF of a person with the disease but not in persons without the disease—in other words, a diagnostic test. For Alzheimer's disease an ideal biomarker would be able to detect a fundamental feature of Alzheimer's neuropathology at an early, preferably pre-symptomatic, phase of the illness, in a manner that would reliably allow Alzheimer cases to be distinguished from other types of dementia as well as from persons without dementia. Such a test needs to be simple, inexpensive and non-invasive. In today's terms this would mean a blood or urine test rather than a test of CSF (which requires an uncomfortable lumbar puncture procedure), though some new types of brain scan may offer an alternative approach.[1]

Diagnostic blood tests

There are divergent views on whether reliable, accurate diagnostic blood tests are likely to be developed. Michael Woodward, a geriatrician from Melbourne and chair of the Australasian Consortium for Clinical Cognitive Research, is optimistic; he believes that by 2007 there will be a range of blood tests available that will be used in combination, with diagnosis depending on a pattern or ratio among a range of biomarkers rather than on a single test. These biomarkers will include blood levels of tau protein, A-beta protein and amyloid percursor protein (APP). For cases where these tests in combination are not sufficiently diagnostic, CSF levels might be used.

Others, such as Henry Brodaty, Professor of Psychogeriatrics at the University of New South Wales in Sydney and chair of Alzheimer's Disease International, and Simon Lovestone, Professor of Old Age Psychiatry at the Institute of Psychiatry in London, are not so sure that these tests will be helpful in diagnosis; they believe that we will find out within the next five to ten years, and that if they prove unsuccessful it is unlikely that such tests will ever be clinically available. As pointed out by Simon Lovestone and Colin Masters, Professor of Pathology at the University of Melbourne, it is already possible to obtain CSF levels of proteins associated with Alzheimer's disease, such as tau and A-beta protein, and that these are not very helpful to a clinician; a recent report, however, found that altered levels of these proteins predicted which individuals with age-related memory impairment would progress to Alzheimer's disease over an eighteen-month period.[2] Others, including Perminder Sachdev, Professor of Neuropsychiatry at the University of New South Wales, Gary Small, Parlow-Solomon Professor on Ageing at UCLA in the United States, and Brian Lawlor, Professor of Psychiatry for the Elderly, Trinity College Dublin, Republic of Ireland, believe that it is unlikely that these blood tests will ever be sufficiently discriminating to be used as diagnostic tests.

Undoubtedly many new blood tests are on the horizon and will be touted by their commercial backers as the 'Alzheimer's test'. The concern is that none will be sufficiently accurate or reliable, and that many people, including doctors, may be misled and thus make inappropriate diagnoses, which could cause considerable anxiety in the general public. David Ames, Associate Professor of Psychiatry of Old Age at the University of Melbourne and the editor of *International Psychogeriatrics*, states that for the foreseeable future a clinical diagnosis based on the presence of the classical presenting syndrome and history, in the absence of confounding diagnoses, will remain the nearest thing to a 'gold standard' that we have.

On the other hand, while these blood tests may not be sufficiently reliable to distinguish Alzheimer's disease from other dementias or from normality, they may be useful to monitor the progress of the condition and to confirm whether new drug treatments were working. Simon Lovestone feels that workable versions would not be available before 2007.

Brain scans

Many dementia experts believe that neuro-imaging, the visualisation of brain structure and/or function by various scanning techniques, will be a more fruitful avenue for early diagnosis than blood tests. There are many different types of brain scans. Most of those routinely available, such as CT and MRI scans, provide images of brain structure and, as described in Chapter 6, are very helpful in assisting with diagnosis; as stand-alone tests, however, they cannot provide a dementia diagnosis. Efforts are now underway to create computerised brain atlases of various diseases that might allow a single CT or MRI scan to be compared with known patterns of disease abnormality. Thus, a brain scan of a person with mild memory problems might reveal a brain pattern consistent with, perhaps, early Alzheimer's disease or simply normal ageing. Although this would be helpful, the analysis of changes over time would be more important. Currently, serial CT or MRI scans over a period of a year or two can detect progressive atrophy or increasing vascular lesions, but they need to be interpreted in conjunction with the 'gold standard' clinical examination. It is now proposed that dynamic (4-D) brain maps will evolve with the design of mathematical systems to track anatomical changes over time and map dynamic patterns of brain degeneration associated with different illnesses.[3] One of the main advantages of such approaches over the methods described below is that CT and, to a lesser extent, MRI scans are reasonably accessible, affordable, safe and tolerable for older people.

Dementia is a clinical syndrome defined by brain function, so it is not surprising that scans of brain function are felt by many researchers to hold out the greatest promise for early, reliable diagnosis. Various types of brain scan that measure aspects of brain function have been available for some years, but for the most part have not achieved sufficient accuracy or reliability to be used other than as a research tool. This is rapidly changing. According to Gary Small, positron emission tomography (PET) scans are now about 90 to 95 per cent accurate (depending on disease severity; they are less accurate in early dementia). PET scans involve the measurement of brain glucose metabolism as a marker of brain function by measuring the uptake of a form of radioactive glucose in various parts of the brain. PET studies have shown reduced activity in the parietal, temporal and pre-frontal lobes of the brain in Alzheimer patients and in the frontal and temporal brain regions in persons with frontotemporal dementia.

There has also been research targeting individuals at high risk of Alzheimer's disease. PET studies in middle-aged persons with the E4 allele of the apoE gene but no dementia have shown a similar pattern of changes to those found in persons with Alzheimer's disease, implying that they are already showing possible early changes of brain function. More subtle abnormalities of function can be detected by comparing scans taken at mental rest and during a brain activation task.[4] One particularly exciting development is PET's ability to detect amyloid plaques, thus measuring the fundamental neuropathological abnormality of Alzheimer's disease. If this finding can be confirmed in much larger studies, it may be possible to use PET scans in non-symptomatic individuals to detect abnormal levels of plaque and tangle accumulation, to assist in the diagnosis of the type of dementia and to monitor the progress of treatment.[5] Such applications may be available in three to five years.

PET scans have a number of disadvantages, however. They involve the use of radioactive isotopes, albeit in small amounts, which requires access to a cyclotron, and there are very few PET facilities available. It seems unlikely that many more will be developed, so they are not going to be routinely available to the general public, although some teaching hospitals might have access to them. PET scans are also reasonably time consuming to perform, require a relatively cooperative subject and are expensive. For all these reasons I doubt whether PET scans will have a major impact in the routine detection and management of dementia, especially as there are other promising alternatives.

Functional MRI (fMRI) scanning is one such alternative. This technique allows the study of brain function and structure simultaneously without exposure to radiation and in less time than PET scanning. Studies have shown that middle-aged persons at high risk of Alzheimer's disease, due to carrying the E4 allele of the apoE gene, have different patterns of activation in the areas of the brain affected by Alzheimer's disease during a memory activation task than individuals not carrying the E4 allele.[6] These changes also predicted decline in memory function over two years. As fMRI is a newer technique than PET scanning, much more data will be required before its potential usefulness in routine clinical practice can be determined. It seems promising in the investigation of pre-symptomatic individuals at high genetic risk and is potentially more accessible than PET scanning, but its use is probably five to ten years off.

The technique of magnetic resonance spectroscopy (MRS) makes it possible to examine biochemical changes in the brain and relate them to behaviour and function. As drug treatments for dementia are primarily aimed at altering levels of neurotransmitters in the brain, the biochemical changes detectable by this technique could become a measure of treatment effect. It is debatable at this stage whether MRS will be clinically useful.

Brain function

A number of studies have shown that smell perception changes in the very early stages of most people with Alzheimer's disease. Intriguingly, a review of the literature has found that odour identification tests are more likely to predict the development of Alzheimer's disease in currently normal individuals than either neuropsychological testing or neuro-imaging. This might suggest a role for such tests in a broadly based screening strategy.

Many of the tests of cognitive function now available, both brief screening tests and more detailed neuropsychological tests, have been shown to be predictive of future cognitive decline in persons with mild cognitive changes, but not to the extent that an accurate diagnosis can be made without serial testing. Brief cognitive tests are not very suitable for serial testing of mild impairment, while repeated full neuropsychological assessments are time consuming, expensive and impractical if considered on a large scale.

A possible alternative, developed in Australia by David Darby, a behavioural neurologist from Victoria, is CogState™, a computer-based test designed to measure cognitive performance in about fifteen to eighteen minutes. It is available over the Internet and can be downloaded free, though interpretation of test results attracts a fee. CogState™ measures objective speed and accuracy in a card game format, which minimises issues related to culture or language. Individual test results have little meaning unless significantly abnormal. It has been designed specifically for multiple testing, as the intended use is to monitor the progress of individuals over time by comparing later test results with baseline tests. Any significant declines over time are highlighted and recommendations made for a full medical review.[7]

There are a number of concerns with this and other similar tests. It remains unproven whether the technique's detection of decline in cognitive function is an accurate predictor of dementia. It also targets the 'worried well' who are searching for reassurance, which may or may not be provided. As any change detected would require full medical and psychiatric evaluation to determine the cause and its significance, it is likely that very often diagnostic uncertainty will remain and a further full evaluation twelve or more months down the track will be required. While this is a promising approach, I cannot recommend its use at this stage until much more research has been independently conducted.

Overall, it seems that in the foreseeable future early diagnosis will involve the monitoring of high risk individuals—for example, those with genetic risk factors, multiple vascular risk factors, impaired smell perception, or mild cognitive changes—from the age of 50 years. Monitoring may involve a screen of blood tests to detect biomarkers of Alzheimer's disease, serial brain scans and serial tests of cognitive function. A combination of these tests may indicate the likelihood that the individual has pre-symptomatic or mildly symptomatic dementia, especially Alzheimer's disease. Such findings will only be useful if effective preventive and treatment strategies are available.

PREVENTION

As described in Chapters 2 and 3, multiple risk factors for Alzheimer's disease and vascular dementia have now been identified, so theoretically it should be possible to prevent dementia in the near future. Indeed, it is suggested that this may be possible within the next ten or fifteen years, say by 2017. In the case of Alzheimer's disease there is general agreement that interventions that prevent amyloid plaque formation will be the cornerstone of therapy, and that the agents involved will be those now used to treat symptomatic Alzheimer's disease. Both Simon Lovestone and Gary Small feel that these agents may also prevent some of the other degenerative dementias. Perminder Sachdev and Michael Woodward stress the importance of attending to other risk factors as well, and are of the opinion that even with this combination of approaches prevention may still be a matter of delay rather than eradication. Brian Lawlor and Michael Woodward feel that delay in the onset of Alzheimer's disease might be reasonably achieved by attention to vascular risk factors alone, such as control of hypertension, cessation of smoking and the use of statin medication, and that the effectiveness of these strategies will become clearer within five years. Colin Masters, in similar fashion, feels that vascular dementia could theoretically be completely prevented by targeting vascular risk factors, though others are sceptical that this would be practically achievable.

One of the main challenges facing this field is to obtain sufficient evidence about different interventions to determine their effectiveness in dementia prevention, whether by delay or by eradication. While effective preventive strategies may well become available over the next ten to fifteen years, it will take much longer than that to evaluate their degree of effectiveness and the relative merits of different interventions and combinations of interventions. It is also clear that despite the wide range of dementia risk factors identified in recent years, the main hopes of Alzheimer's disease prevention rest in the development of new drugs that target the accumulation of amyloid. In other words, attention to the other risk factors alone may have only limited benefit.

TREATMENT

More effective disease modifying treatments projected for symptomatic Alzheimer's disease will prevent amyloid plaque formation by interfering with the amyloid cascade. A number of other types of treatments could also work.

Secretase inhibitors

There are a number of drugs being developed in this category, with at least one having completed Phase II trials. They work by reducing the production of beta-amyloid protein.

Beta-amyloid vaccination

Immunisation (vaccination) aims to increase the cleavage (break-down) of beta-amyloid protein through a number of approaches that all involve the production of antibodies.

Such treatment is likely to be used in combination with other therapies, some of which are currently available but unproven— for example, statins that reduce cholesterol, anti-inflammatory drugs, control of blood pressure in midlife, antioxidants such as vitamins C and E, and folic acid, along with lifestyle changes to diet (low in fat; high in grains, greens and fish), optimal alcohol consumption (about two glasses of red wine per day), physical and mental exercise, avoidance of head injuries and no smoking. These treatments are also likely to be beneficial for vascular dementia, mixed vascular/Alzheimer's dementia and dementia with Lewy bodies, though the degree of benefit is uncertain.

Two exciting treatments that may ultimately become important components of therapy are gene therapy and foetal stem cell grafts. The potentials are enormous, though there are many scientific, ethical and logistical hurdles to jump before they can be used. If a 'cure' for Alzheimer's disease and other degenerative dementias is ever developed, it is likely to involve one of these therapies, but it may well be at least 20, if not 50, years away.

Gene therapy

In 2001, the first two-year study to test the safety of gene therapy in Alzheimer's disease was commenced in San Diego. It involves eight patients with mild Alzheimer's disease. In this study, fibro-blast cells obtained from the skin of the patients are cultured and then genetically modified in a test tube to produce and secrete the human nerve growth factor (NGF) molecule. The patients receive intracerebral injections of their own fibroblasts into the regions of their brains where neurons are undergoing atrophy as a result of Alzheimer's disease. The eventual goal is to determine whether NGF produced by the cells implanted into the brain can prevent the death of some of the nerve cells affected by the Alzheimer's disease, and enhance the function of some of the remaining brain cells. If this study is successful, gene therapy may be used in the future in combination with drugs that prevent amyloid plaque formation. The drugs will stop further damage from occurring while the gene therapy will attempt to restore neurons that have already perished.[8]

Stem cell grafts

This is a very controversial topic, as evidenced by the impassioned debates that took place in Federal Parliament about the use of foetal stem cells before enabling legislation was passed in December 2002. A stem cell is an unspecialised cell that has the ability to renew itself indefinitely. Under appropriate conditions it can give rise to a wide range of mature cell types in the human body. Any disorder that involves loss of or injury to normal cells is a candidate for stem cell therapy. In this regard, many disorders of the nervous system, including Alzheimer's disease, Parkinson's disease and the other degenerative dementias, are prime targets for neuronal stem cell therapy.[9]

Stem cells can be obtained from a variety of sources, including embryos, foetal tissue and some adult tissues. At this stage in animal experiments, adult neuronal stem cells have not been shown to form neurones though foetal neuronal stem cells do. Hence the current debate and the importance of this particular type of stem cell. It is possible that other types of stem cells may eventually be found that will form neurones.

How would stem cell therapy work in dementia? There are two general approaches. The first involves the transplantation of undifferentiated (immature) cells whose subsequent development would be controlled by cues derived from the patient's brain. The use of the second approach is more likely; in this method stem cells are grown in a culture dish into the desired type of neurone according to the disease being treated—thus the cells grown for Parkinson's disease would be different from those grown for Alzheimer's disease. These cells would be transplanted back into the brain of the person being treated as a neuronal graft. This approach requires a greater understanding than we yet have of how to culture stem cells into the desired cell type.

To date, most work in this field has involved the treatment of Parkinson's disease and overall the results have been moderately encouraging, with no major risks emerging. There are still many unknowns to be resolved, including long-term cell survival, risks of immunological rejection and, not least, logistical issues about supply of tissue and ethical concerns. It is likely to be at least 20 years before we know whether stem cell therapy will be viable in the treatment of Alzheimer's disease. If it does work, it will probably be used in combination with drug treatments in a similar fashion to gene therapy.

There are many other treatments currently in varying stages of investigation that often feature in media reports. Some may have great potential, others will probably have a limited effect or may never demonstrate sufficient benefit or safety for clinical use.[10] These are listed in Table 13.1. One that deserves extra comment is clioquinol. This is an old drug, formerly marketed to treat amoebic infections, which is now being investigated by Colin Masters in Melbourne. It prevents the accumulation of amyloid by chelating (removing) copper and zinc, which in turn inhibits amyloid-forming enzymes. It may also promote the dissolution and clearance of amyloid from the brain. Some early Australian clinical trials have shown a limited effect and more detailed evaluation is required.

A fantastical notion, raised by Henry Brodaty, is the possibility of downloading our memories onto a microchip so that, if dementia set in, we could upload them again once the disease process was stabilised. If we can have bionic ears and prosthetic limbs, why not a prosthetic memory? Seems to be the basis for a science fiction story!

HOW WILL EFFECTIVE PREVENTION AND TREATMENT OF DEMENTIA AFFECT SOCIETY?

The demographic imperative of an ageing society that has driven much of the research into various aspects of dementia care from a molecular to a societal level was discussed in Chapter 1. Based on projections of population growth, the number of dementia cases in Australia is predicted to increase from around 165 000 in 2003 to 459 000 in 2041. But what will it mean for society if, by 2041, effective dementia therapies can prevent the onset of dementia, halt the progression of early dementia, and possibly reverse some, if not all, of the damage done to come close to a 'cure'? If dementia is largely removed as the main cause of disability in older

Table 13.1 Summary of new treatments for Alzheimer's disease

Treatment	How it works	Potential effectiveness	Potential drawbacks	When available
Secretase inhibitors	Reduce the production of beta-amyloid protein	Very effective; may halt the damage and result in improvement	Unknown at present but likely to have significant side-effects	10–15 years
Beta-amyloid vaccination	Increases the breakdown of beta-amyloid protein	Very effective; may halt the damage and result in improvement	Brain haemorrhage, immune reactions	10–15 years
Gene therapy	Genetically modified cells implanted in the brain to stimulate nerve growth	Very effective; will replace damaged and dead cells; used with drugs that halt disease process	Unknown at present but could include brain haemorrhage, tumour formation, chronic pain and weight loss	20+ years
Stem cell neuronal grafts	Stem cells cultured to form specific neuronal cells deficient in Alzheimer's disease are implanted in the brain as a neuronal graft	Very effective; will replace damaged and dead cells; used with drugs that halt disease process	Unknown at present but could include brain haemorrhage, tumour formation	20+ years
GSK inhibitors	Reduce the production of amyloid and tau protein	Very effective; may halt the damage and result in improvement	Unknown at present but likely to have significant side-effects	10–20 years

continues . . .

Table 13.1 Summary of new treatments for Alzheimer's disease (continued)

Treatment	How it works	Potential effectiveness	Potential drawbacks	When available
Phenserine	Cholinesterase inhibitor (CHEI) that might affect amyloid production	Moderately effective; depends upon the effects on amyloid	Gastrointestinal and other side-effects found in CHEIs	5 years
CPHPC	Reduces serum amyloid protein blood levels and may reduce amyloid plaque formation, but this is unproven	Very effective; may halt the damage and result in improvement	Unknown at present; early trials reveal no major problems	10–20 years
Colostrinin	An antioxidant extracted from the milk of ewes after they have given birth; may prevent the formation of or dissolve amyloid plaques	Moderately effective; early studies show limited benefit; for use in combination therapy	Sleeplessness	5–10 years
Clioquinol	Prevents the accumulation of amyloid by removing copper and zinc, which in turn inhibits amyloid-forming enzymes	Moderately effective; early studies show limited benefit; for use in combination therapy	Appears well tolerated in early Australian trials	5–10 years

COGNIShunt	A pump implanted in the brain removes CSF to prevent toxic proteins from accumulating and forming plaques and tangles	Moderately effective; early studies show limited benefit; not likely to work by itself	Infections of the pump and brain; invasive surgery for moderate benefit	5–10 years
Leteprinim potassium (Neotrofin)	Restores nerve function by repairing and regenerating nerve cells	Moderately effective at best; studies halted in 2002 due to lack of effect	Appears well tolerated	5–10 years
CX516 (Ampalex)	Increases the activity of nerve receptors in the brain that compensate for decreased production of glutamate, an important memory neurotransmitter	Moderately effective in theory, but awaiting data; possibly useful in combination with CHEIs	Currently in Phase II trials for safety and efficacy	5–10 years

Australians, will they live longer in good health or will other serious conditions—cancer, arthritis, heart disease, diabetes, lung disease—simply become more apparent as causes of disability? As dementia is now the main reason for admission to residential care, would there still be the same level of need for these facilities or could we look after even more people in their own homes?

These are all important questions that are not really answerable at present. Some authorities theorise that the natural lifespan for humans may be around 115 to 120 years. Ideally, effective treatments for any illness would allow a person to live their natural lifespan with minimal disability and a good quality of life. But the availability of effective treatments would not necessarily mean that most people for whom they were suitable would use them. This might happen due to cost (none of the new dementia drugs is likely to be cheap), the ignorance of doctors, patients and carers about the availability of treatment, a failure to detect dementia until a late stage (when treatments might have only limited benefit), or the refusal of some people to be treated. An ongoing study from Baltimore in the United States, conducted by Peter Rabins, illustrates these issues. It has found that only about 50 per cent of older people with significant cognitive impairment were recognised by their family as having a memory problem, around 25 per cent were identified by their doctor, and only 14 per cent were being treated with cholinesterase inhibitors. Some of these figures might be reduced through education about dementia, but I suspect that there will always be a significant number of untreated people. Even if one-third of the potential cases of dementia in 2041 were to be treated (and I believe that proportion is optimistic), that would still leave around 150 000 untreated cases, approximately the number of people with dementia in Australia in 2002!

If diagnostic problems were to be overcome and most people with dementia were to receive effective treatment, the inbuilt assumption is that they will die of other serious conditions. As implied in Chapter 1, there is a flaw in that argument. This is the tendency to ignore the rapid progress occurring in the prevention and treatment of most major medical conditions. In other words, older people are likely to potentially reduce their risks of succumbing to a whole range of potentially terminal illnesses. But—effective treatments for other serious disabling, but not terminal, conditions of old age, such as blindness from macular degeneration, nerve deafness, immobility from osteoarthritis and other causes of frailty, may not be discovered during the same time frame as a treatment for dementia. This could result in an increasing population of alert but frail, disabled and possibly demoralised older people who feel trapped by their incapacities.

Another possibility is that the new dementia treatments may not work indefinitely and may simply end up delaying the dementia for five to ten years. Does this mean that older people will die of other conditions before the dementia takes effect—a bit like it used to be 50 years ago? This may not be the case. We may delay the dementia, allowing people to live a longer, healthier life until the dementia symptoms start to occur at an older age.

SUMMARY

There are many exciting developments ahead in the prevention and treatment of dementia in general and Alzheimer's disease in particular. While this augurs well for the future, it is unlikely that any cures will become available for at least 20 years, and likely that many of those treated will remain disabled with significant impairments. Despite the improvements, the number of older people in Australia with dementia will still increase over the next 20 or 30 years at least. Family carers will remain their primary source of support, even though the number of family carers potentially available will diminish in the same time period due to Australia's declining fertility and marital rates. Thus for the foreseeable future, systems similar to those currently in place to support dementing people and their carers will remain the cornerstone of dementia care in Australia.

Appendix 1

Australian telephone helplines

Most of these numbers are only available in Australia and the 1800 numbers are free except for mobile phones where mobile rates apply.

Alzheimer's Association Dementia Helpline
1800 639 331

Carers Australia
Information and support 1800 242 636

Commonwealth Carelink Centres
Commonwealth Government helpline with information for carers 1800 052 222

Aged and Community Care Information Line
Commonwealth Government helpline with information about Aged Care Assessment Teams, community services and residential services 1800 500 853

Department of Veterans' Affairs
Commonwealth Government helpline for veterans and their families 1800 555 254

Advocare
An advocacy service for disabled people   1800 655 566

NSW Office of the Public Guardian
For urgent decisions for a disabled person in New South Wales who has had a public guardian appointed by the Guardianship Tribunal 1800 451 510

NSW Guardianship Tribunal
For applications for a guardian to be appointed in New South Wales
1800 463 928

Victorian and Civil Administrative Tribunal—Guardianship List
For guardianship applications in Victoria 1800 133 055

Office of the Public Advocate (South Australia)
For guardianship issues in South Australia 1800 066 969

Guardianship and Administration Board (Tasmania)
(03) 6233 3085

Guardianship, Administration and Advocacy (Western Australia)
1800 191 009

Office of the Public Advocate (Queensland)
07 3224 7424

Appendix 2

Websites

Australia

Government

Ageing and Aged Care Division, Australian Department of Health and Ageing
http://www.health.gov.au/acc/index.htm
This is the Australian Government website that provides information about residential and community aged care services in Australia. Specifically, apart from describing the services, it gives detailed information about the various eligibility criteria for different services, from the perspectives of older people, carers and service providers. It is regularly updated so the information is almost certainly accurate at the time of accessing. There is also information about dementia and the Australian Government policy for dementia. Links to State health departments are also present.

Lists of Aged Care Services in Australia, Australian Department of Health and Ageing
http://www.health.gov.au/acc/rescare/servlist/servlist.htm
If you want to find out how to contact your local aged care service, this is the place to go.

Lists of Aged Care Assessment Teams, Australian Department of Health and Ageing
http://www.health.gov.au/acc/contacts/acat/acatindx.htm
This is where you find out how to contact your local Aged Care Assessment Team.

Commonwealth Carelink Centres
http://www.health.gov.au/acc/cclinkc/index.htm
This is the Australian Government site about Commonwealth Carelink

Centres that allow Australians to access information about community and other aged care services, with a single phone call or visit to a Commonwealth Carelink Centre shopfront.

Australian Institute of Health and Welfare
http://www.aihw.gov.au/
This is Australia's national agency for health and welfare statistics and information. It contains many reports on ageing, including the excellent *Older Australians at a Glance*. There is also much statistical information about residential and community aged care, dementia and carers.

Health Insurance Commission
http://www.hic.gov.au/
This site provides helpful consumer information about Medicare, including how to make claims and get replacement Medicare cards, and the Medicare safety-net scheme. It is also the site to get information about the Pharmaceutical Benefits Scheme (PBS).

Non-government

Alzheimer's Australia
http://www.alzheimers.org.au/
This is the website of the Alzheimer's Association Australia, which represents at the national level the interests of its federation of State and Territory members on all matters relating to dementia and carer issues in Australia. Excellent 'Help Sheets' for carers (prepared by the Victorian branch) about many aspects of dementia and its management are available for downloading. There are also some well thought out policy documents and commentaries. You can also obtain information about how to contact your local branch, and about national and international conferences.

Carers Australia
http://www.carersaustralia.com.au/
Carers Australia represents the needs and interests of carers and their families, irrespective of the type of physical, mental or intellectual disability of the cared-for person. The website provides information about the policy statements and public advocacy of the organisation. There is also information about the recently introduced Medicines Line, the first national telephone service of its kind in Australia, helping the public make sense of their medicines through access, quality evidence and independent information. Information about how to obtain information and support is provided.

Council on the Ageing
http://www.cota.org.au/
The Council on the Ageing (COTA) is the peak consumer organisation dedicated to protecting and promoting the well-being of older people in Australia. Its website provides a plethora of information about all matters relating to ageing including COTA's submissions on policy issues as diverse as broadband Internet and healthcare. There is also a wonderful page containing fact sheets for consumers about all matters pertaining to ageing and aged care in Australia. COTA is also involved in the publication of the *Australasian Journal on Ageing* and information about this and other COTA publications is available on the website.

Aged and Community Services Australia
http://www.agedcare.org.au/
This is the website of the national peak body in Australia representing over 1400 church and charitable organisations providing accommodation and community care services to older people. The website includes fact sheets about residential care, dementia, carers, community care, health, Medicare and the ageing of Australia. Information about policies, projects, publications and conferences is also provided.

Advocare
http://members.iinet.net.au/~advocare/
Advocare is an independent Australian advocacy service that promotes the rights and best interests of people receiving aged residential and community care services, and of those people who are not receiving services but are entitled to them.

Australian Society for Geriatric Medicine (ASGM)
http://www.asgm.org.au/
The ASGM is the peak organisation in Australia for geriatricians. The website has policy statements about a range of issues with a medical focus on aged care in Australia.

The Australian Association of Gerontology
http://www.aag.asn.au/
The Australian Association of Gerontology has the mission to expand the knowledge of ageing through research, education, networking and policy development. On its website is an Educational Guide to courses on ageing and age-related conditions in Australia, and information about conferences.

Australasian Consortium for Clinical Cognitive Research (AC4R)
http://www.med.unsw.edu.au/ac4r/
This is the website that brings together Australian and New Zealand clinicians involved in clinical research, particularly drug trials, in dementia.

The Royal Australian and New Zealand College of Psychiatrists
http://www.ranzcp.org/
The resource section on this site is a gateway to information about a range of mental health matters. The Faculty of Psychiatry of Old Age also has a page.

Aged Care Standards and Accreditation Agency
http://www.accreditation.aust.com/index.html
The Aged Care Standards and Accreditation Agency is the independent body responsible for managing the accreditation process and ongoing supervision and support for aged care homes in Australia. On this site you can access inspection reports about individual aged care homes.

Rights of Older People
http://www.agedrights.asn.au/home.html
This website provides information about the nationwide network of advocacy services, and about the ways that advocacy services can assist older people (or their representatives).

National Aged Care Alliance
http://www.naca.asn.au/
The National Aged Care Alliance is a representative body of peak national organisations in aged care, including consumer groups, providers, unions and health professionals, working together to determine a more positive future for aged care in Australia.

National Ageing Research Institute
http://www.mednwh.unimelb.edu.au/ageingwell.html
This research institute is located in Melbourne and its website has some good consumer information about ageing and age-related medical conditions, including dementia.

Australian Nursing Home and Extended Care Association
http://www.anheca.com.au/
ANHECA exists to promote the interests of private, church and charitably run nursing homes and hostels within Australia, so that they may deliver high standards of care.

CogState
http://www.cogstate.com/
This is a computerised test of cognitive function available over the Internet that can be accessed by the general public for a fee. The test is repeated over time and is alleged to be sensitive to early cognitive decline, though it cannot distinguish the cause. A test for the 'worried well' with plenty of money.

NSW Office of the Public Guardian
http://www.lawlink.nsw.gov.au/opg.nsf/pages/index
Information about guardianship, enduring guardianship and substitute consent in New South Wales.

NSW Guardianship Tribunal
http://www.gt.nsw.gov.au
Information about how to apply for a guardianship order in New South Wales, and links to sites that contain relevant New South Wales legislation.

Victorian Civil and Administrative Tribunal (VCAT)
http://www.vcat.vic.gov.au/
In 1998, VCAT took over the administration of the guardianship list in Victoria.

The Public Advocate (Queensland)
http://www.justice.qld.gov.au/guardian/pa.htm
Information is available on adult guardianship and power of attorney in Queensland.

Office of the Public Advocate (South Australia)
http://www.opa.sa.gov.au/index.htm
Information is available on the Guardianship Board in South Australia.

Guardianship and Administration Board (Tasmania)
http://www.justice.tas.gov.au/guar/index.htm
Information is available about guardianship and the public guardian in Tasmania.

Guardianship, Administration and Advocacy (Western Australia)
http://www.justice.wa.gov.au
Information is available about guardianship, advocacy and enduring power of attorney in Western Australia.

INTERNATIONAL

Alzheimer's Disease Education and Referral (ADEAR) Center
http://www.alzheimers.org/
This is a service of the US National Institute on Aging (NIA), one of the National Institutes of Health in the USA. The purpose of the website is to provide information about Alzheimer's disease and related disorders. It publicises recent research findings and has an email service to notify all registrants of new information. Multimedia educational material is available for lay people, clinicians and academics. You can even pose questions to NIA experts and receive a personal email reply. Other information

available includes a large, recently revised bibliography, a list of current research trials in dementia and links to other worthwhile sites. While this site has an American focus, the quality of the general information about dementia is outstanding.

Alzheimer's Disease International
http://www.alz.co.uk/
Alzheimer's Disease International is the umbrella organisation of Alzheimer associations around the world, which offer support and information to people with dementia and their carers. The website provides information about Alzheimer's disease, the global impact of Alzheimer's disease and how to find help. It also has a Cross Cultural Dementia Network that collates details of organisations that work with ethnic communities, rural populations, refugees and people of different sexual orientation.

Alzheimer's Association (USA)
http://www.alz.org/
This is the website of the US Alzheimer's Association. On this site you'll find information about the disease as well as about the Association's efforts in the USA. An interesting page contains balanced information about alternative therapies.

Alzheimer's Society: Dementia care and research
http://www.alzheimers.org.uk/index.html
This is the UK Alzheimer's Society website. It has a very good range of help sheets about various aspects of dementia that can be downloaded.

US Administration on Aging Alzheimer's Resource Room
http://www.aoa.dhhs.gov/alz/index.asp
The US Administration on Aging's resource 'room' website provides families, carers and professionals with information about Alzheimer's disease, caregiving, working with and providing services to persons with Alzheimer's.

The Whole Brain Atlas
http://www.med.harvard.edu/AANLIB/
This Harvard Medical School website has CT scan, MRI scan and SPECT scan images of a wide range of neurological disorders, as well as normal ageing. There is a guided tour on the Alzheimer brain.

The Alzheimer's Foundation (NZ)
http://www.alzheimers.co.nz/
The Alzheimer's Foundation was established in New Zealand in 1985 to provide support for carers of people with Alzheimer's disease. The website provides practical information about community and residential

care services in New Zealand, as well as other information about dementia, support groups and education.

Alzheimer's New Zealand Inc.
http://www.alzheimers.org.nz/
Alzheimer's New Zealand Inc. is a charitable organisation and the national body for 22 Alzheimer's member organisations located throughout the country. The website contains practical information about dementia with a New Zealand focus.

American Association for Geriatric Psychiatry
http://www.aagpgpa.org/p_c/default.asp
This is the website for American psychiatrists who specialise in treating older people. It has an excellent page with consumer information about dementia and depression in old age. There are Spanish language versions as well.

International Psychogeriatric Association
http://www.ipa-online.org/ipaonlinev3/home/default.asp
This is the peak international organisation for psychiatrists and other mental health professionals who treat older people. The website has an excellent section about the behavioural and psychological symptoms of dementia.

MEDLINEplus—Alzheimer's disease
http://www.nlm.nih.gov/medlineplus/alzheimersdisease.html
This site from the US National Library of Medicine has links to the most recent research findings about Alzheimer's disease as well as to other important American sites that contain information for consumers and health professionals.

Mayo Clinic Alzheimer's Center
http://www.mayoclinic.com/findinformation/conditioncenters/centers/
This world-famous medical clinic in Rochester, Minnesota, in the USA has one of the best health websites on the net; its Alzheimer's Center page is excellent. It is full of accessible information and good practical tips. There is also a good page that covers the topic of communicating with children about Alzheimer's disease.

National Institute of Neurological Disorders and Stroke— Alzheimer's disease information page
http://www.ninds.nih.gov/health_and_medical/disorders/
alzheimersdisease_doc.htm
Another major American health institute that has an excellent site with mainly medical information about Alzheimer's disease. On another page

is a very informative description of the life and death of neurons that can be downloaded in full colour.

American Geriatrics Society
http://www.healthinaging.org/public_education/pef/
The American Geriatrics Society website has an excellent page dedicated to public education with recent information on topics that include dementia, caregiving, over-the-counter drugs, swallowing problems, incontinence, advance directives, persistent pain and many more.

The Merck Manual of Geriatrics
http://www.merck.com/pubs/mm_geriatrics/home.html
If you want some quick information about medical problems in old age, this is a good place to start.

The New Zealand Geriatrics Society (NZGS)
http://www.nzgs.org.nz/index.html
The NZGS is the peak organisation in New Zealand for geriatricians.

Lewy-net. Dementia with Lewy bodies
http://www.nottingham.ac.uk/pathology/lewy/lewyhome.html
Everything you want to know about dementia with Lewy bodies.

The Huntington's Disease Society of America
http://www.hdsa.org/edu/edu.html
Information on the genetic disorder Huntington's disease.

Appendix 3

Books for carers

Early Stage Dementia—Lorraine West, Gill and Macmillan Ltd, Dublin, 2003
This Australian book seeks to support and guide individuals, families and professionals as they begin a journey with dementia.

The 36-Hour Day: A Family Guide to Caring for Persons with Alzheimer's Disease, Related Dementing Illnesses, and Memory Loss in Later Life (3rd edn)—Nancy Mace and Peter Rabins, Johns Hopkins University Press, Baltimore, 1999
This is the classic book for dementia carers and provides support, factual information and practical tips.

Dementia with Dignity (2nd edn)—Barbara Sherman, McGraw-Hill Professional, Sydney, 2000
This Australian book is a guide for family and professional dementia carers.

Communication and the Care of People with Dementia—John Killick and Kate Allan, Open University Press, Maidenhead, UK, 2001
This book argues that communication is at the heart of all approaches to dementia care, and is an in-depth exploration of ways of establishing and developing communication with people with dementia.

Dementia: Alzheimer's and Other Dementias—Harry Cayton, Nori Graham and James Warner, Class Publishing, London, 2002
This British guide for carers provides the answers for many commonly posed questions.

The Validation Training Program: the Practice of Validation—Evelyn Sutton and Naomi Feil, Health Professions Press, Baltimore, 1999
This is a manual for validation therapy.

The Carer Experience: Information and Ideas for Carers of People with Dementia—Commonwealth Department of Health and Family Services, AGPS, Canberra, 2002
This Australian book has a section on ways carers can look after themselves.

GLOSSARY

acetylcholine A neurotransmitter involved in learning and memory that is severely diminished in Alzheimer's disease.

activities of daily living (ADL) Personal care activities necessary for everyday living, such as eating, bathing, grooming, dressing and toileting.

advance directives (living wills) Written statements made by a competent person about what medical treatment they would like when they are no longer competent to make the decision.

advocate A person who acts on behalf of another party.

age-associated memory impairment A decline in short-term memory that sometimes accompanies ageing.

Aged Care Assessment Team (ACAT) A multidisciplinary team that performs comprehensive assessments of the needs of older people and people with disabilities.

Aged Care Client Record The form completed by an ACAT that allows access to certain community services and residential care.

ageing in place An approach that aims to provide residents with appropriate care and increased choice by allowing them to remain in the same aged care home regardless of their levels of care needs.

alpha-synuclein Protein found in Lewy bodies; occurs in dementia with Lewy bodies and Parkinson's disease.

Alzheimer's disease The most common type of dementia amongst older people.

amnestic disorders A group of disorders characterised by loss of memory in the absence of other cortical dysfunction.

amyloid plaque Insoluble clumps of beta-amyloid protein found in the brains of people with Alzheimer's disease.

amyloid precursor protein (APP) A large protein from which beta-amyloid is derived; found throughout the brain.

antioxidants Substances that remove free radicals which are thought to damage the brain.

aphasia Loss of language skills that can involve comprehension (receptive aphasia), ability to use language (expressive aphasia) or both.

apolipoprotein E (apoE) A protein synthesised in the liver and brain that is involved in lipid metabolism and found to be associated with Alzheimer's disease.

atrophy Shrinkage, usually due to nerve cell death when it occurs in the brain.

autonomy A person's right to make decisions for themselves.

behaviour management Therapy targeted at specific behaviours in an attempt to extinguish unwanted behaviour and encourage desired behaviour.

behavioural and psychological symptoms of dementia (BPSD) Symptoms of dementia that include mood disorders, psychosis, wandering, disruptive vocalisation, aggression and agitation.

beta-amyloid protein The protein that accumulates in amyloid plaques in people with Alzheimer's disease.

BPSD (*see* **behavioural and psychological symptoms of dementia**)

brahmi A popular Indian herb used to treat a range of nervous complaints, including memory loss.

carer or caregiver A person who looks after or gives care to a disabled person.

central nervous system (CNS) The brain and spinal cord.

cerebral haemorrhage Stroke due to bleeding into the brain.

cerebral infarction Stroke due to loss of blood supply to the brain.

cerebrospinal fluid (CSF) Fluid circulating around the brain and spinal cord that contains nutrients and removes toxins.

cholinesterase inhibitors Medications used to treat Alzheimer's disease that increase the availability of acetylcholine in the brain by inhibiting its breakdown.

cognition The mental activities associated with thinking, learning and memory.

Community Aged Care Package (CACP) An integrated package of community care services tailored to meet the needs of an individual.

competency Ability of a person to make rational decisions concerning personal affairs or welfare.

computerised tomography (CT) scan A computerised X-ray that gives a 3-D view of the body.

Creutzfeldt-Jakob disease (CJD) A rare infectious disease that causes dementia.

CT scan (*see* **computerised tomography**)

decision-making capacity To have the capacity to make a decision, the person must be capable of understanding the nature of the decision and the effects that the decision will have upon the person and others.

delirium (acute confusional state)   A transient, global disorder of cognition that develops over days to weeks, usually due to an acute medical problem or medication.

delusion   An unshakeable false belief that is out of keeping with the person's cultural or religious background.

dementia   An acquired decline in memory and thinking (cognition) due to brain disease that results in significant impairment of personal, social or occupational function.

dementia with Lewy bodies   A type of degenerative dementia characterised by fluctuating level of consciousness, parkinsonism and visual hallucinations.

depression   A mental disorder involving a lowering of mood and other negative emotions, loss of interests, reduced activities, sleep, appetite and weight changes.

disorientation   Impairment in the person's awareness of who they are (person), where they are (place) or of when it is (time).

double-blind placebo-controlled study   A research study in which an active treatment is compared with an inactive treatment, and neither the patient nor the therapist knows which treatment is being given.

dysmnestic syndrome   A syndrome characterised by severe impairment of short-term memory without other cognitive changes.

elder abuse   Physical, psychological or financial harm committed against an older person.

enduring power of attorney   A legal document by which a mentally competent person authorises someone to make financial decisions and sign papers on their behalf that contains a statement that this authorisation will continue when their mental capacity is lost.

executive function   The functions of the frontal lobe of the brain.

free radicals   Small molecules that damage the brain in oxidative metabolism.

frontotemporal dementia   A type of degenerative dementia that mainly affects the frontal and temporal lobes of the brain.

gene   Genes are made up of four chemicals arranged in various patterns on the chromosome in the nucleus of each cell; they direct the manufacture of every enzyme, hormone and other protein in the body.

geriatrician   A physician who specialises in treating older people.

guardian   A legally appointed person who is a substitute decision maker for a mentally incompetent person.

hallucination   A perception without a stimulus.

hippocampus   Part of the brain important in memory function.

Home and Community Care (HACC) Services   A program of basic maintenance and support services for frail older people, younger people with disabilities, and the carers of these people, to prevent premature admission to residential care.

Huntington's disease   A hereditary disorder that causes involuntary movements, personality change and dementia.

impairment   Objective weakening, damage or deterioration as a result of injury or disease.

incidence   The number of new cases of a disease in a defined population over a specific period of time.

incontinence   Loss of control of bladder and/or bowel function.

instrumental activities of daily living (IADL)   Higher order activities that include shopping, managing finances, cooking and housework.

magnetic resonance imaging (MRI)   A type of computerised scan that uses strong electromagnetic fields to provide a 3-D image.

memory   The ability to remember past experiences.

memory clinic   A clinic that specialises in the assessment and management of people with disorders of memory.

mild cognitive impairment (MCI)   Mild memory changes, more severe than normal ageing but not sufficient to be regarded as dementia.

Mini-Mental State Examination (MMSE)   A commonly used standardised test of cognitive function.

MRI scan (*see* magnetic resonance imaging)

multidisciplinary team   A clinical team composed of members from different disciplines, such as medicine, nursing, occupational therapy, physical therapy and psychology.

music therapy   A type of therapy that uses music to relieve symptoms of depression, agitation and distress.

neurodegeneration   Progressive degeneration and death of nerve cells.

neurofibrillary tangles   Composed of a protein called tau, and found in nerve cells in Alzheimer's disease and frontotemporal dementia.

neuro-imaging   Brain scans, for example, computerised tomography (CT), magnetic resonance imaging (MRI).

neurologist   A physician who specialises in disorders of the nervous system.

neuron   Nerve cell.

neuropathology   The study of diseases of the nervous system, usually involving microscopic examination.

neuropsychologist   A psychologist with training to perform and interpret standardised tests of cognition and mental functioning.

neurotransmitter   A chemical messenger in the brain.

normal pressure hydrocephalus   A type of dementia caused by blockage in the flow of cerebrospinal fluid (CSF) in the brain resulting in enlarged ventricles.

paranoia   Suspiciousness.

Parkinson's disease   A degenerative disease of the brain that results in slowing of movements, tremor, muscular rigidity and, usually, mental changes.

parkinsonism Slowing of movements, tremor and/or muscular rigidity.

PEG (percutaneous endoscopic gastrostomy) tube A tube placed through the abdominal wall into the stomach to allow tube feeding.

perseveration The constant repetition of a meaningless word or phrase.

pharmacotherapy Drug therapy, medication.

Pick's disease A type of frontotemporal dementia.

placebo An inactive treatment ('sugar pill') used for comparison with a new treatment to see if it works.

placement Transfer of an elderly person to a residential facility such as a nursing home, residential hospital or supervised hostel.

plaques (*see* amyloid plaque)

polypharmacy Prescription of multiple drugs to the same patient with the potential for drug–drug interactions and adverse effects.

power of attorney A legal document by which a mentally competent person authorises someone to make financial decisions and sign papers on their behalf.

prevalence The number of cases of a disease existing in a given population.

prions Small glycoproteins with infectious qualities found in Creutzfeldt-Jakob disease.

progressive supranuclear palsy Rare subcortical dementia involving gaze abnormalities, parkinsonism and unsteady walking.

psychogeriatrician A psychiatrist who specialises in treating older people with mental disorders.

psychosis A mental condition characterised by delusions and/or hallucinations in which the person has lost touch with reality.

psychotropic drugs Drugs used to treat the psychological and behavioural aspects of dementia.

reality orientation A type of therapy used in moderate–severe dementia to improve memory and orientation.

receptor A docking site on a nerve cell where neurotransmitters work.

reminiscence therapy A therapy used in dementia to invoke pleasant life memories, provide distraction and mental stimulation.

respite care Temporary formal care of a person with dementia to give the carer a rest.

risk factors Factors associated with a disease process.

senile dementia An outdated term once used to refer to any form of dementia that occurred in older people.

senility An outdated term that implies that mental deterioration and dementia is a part of normal ageing.

statins Medication used to reduce cholesterol levels that may help in preventing Alzheimer's disease.

subcortical dementia Dementia commencing in or mainly affecting areas of the brain below the cortex, for example, Huntington's disease, Parkinson's disease.

substitute decision maker   The person who makes decisions on behalf of a mentally incompetent person.

sundowning   Agitated behaviour that characteristically occurs in late afternoon and early evening.

support group   A group that provides emotional support to carers.

synapse   The gap between nerve cells where neurotransmitters convey messages between nerves.

tangles (*see* neurofibrillary tangles)

tau protein   The protein found in neurofibrillary tangles.

testamentary capacity   Capacity to make a will.

tube feeding   Use of a feeding tube either through the nose or abdominal wall (*see* **PEG tube**) when a person is unable to swallow safely.

validation therapy   A therapy that assists in communication with moderate–severe dementia by validating the person's emotions.

vascular dementia   A type of dementia due to damage caused by blood vessel disease in the brain.

wandering   A term encompassing several types of behavioural changes found in dementia, including restlessness, aimless walking and goal-directed walking.

NOTES

CHAPTER 1

1 Mathers, C., Vos, T. and Stevenson, C. *The Burden of Disease and Injury in Australia*, AIHW Cat. No. PHE 17, Canberra, 1999, p. 23.

2 Henderson, A.S. and Jorm, A.F. *Dementia in Australia*, Australian Government Publishing Service, Canberra, January, 1998, pp. 5–6.

3 Melding, P. 'The effects of ageing' in P. Melding and B. Draper (eds) *Geriatric Consultation Liaison Psychiatry*, Oxford University Press, Oxford, 2001, pp. 35–56.

4 Brodaty, H. 'Overview of dementia' in *Essentials of Dementia*, Science Press, London, 2001, p. 1.

5 Henderson and Jorm *Dementia in Australia*, pp. 12–13; Australian Bureau of Statistics *Population by Age and Sex, Australian States and Territories*, Cat. No. 3201.0, Commonwealth of Australia, 2001.

6 Henderson and Jorm *Dementia in Australia*, p. 15.

7 ibid., pp. 16–17.

8 World Health Organization *World Health Report 2001*, World Health Organization, Geneva, 2001 http://www.who.int/whr2001/2001/main/en/00library_cat_info.htm [accessed December 3, 2002].

9 Mathers, C., Vos., T. and Stevenson, C. *The Burden of Disease and Injury in Australia*, pp. 25–6.

10 Access Economics, 'The dementia epidemic: economic impact and positive solutions for Australia', Canberra, March 2003, p. 1.

11 ibid., p. 1.

12 Alzheimer's Association (US) *Statistics about Alzheimer's Disease*, http://www.alz.org/AboutAD/Statistics.htm [accessed December 4, 2002].

13 Jorm, A. *Dementia: A Major Health Problem in Australia*, Alzheimer's Association Australia, Position Paper 1, September 2001, p. 3, www.alzheimers.org.au [accessed December 3, 2002].

CHAPTER 2

1   Alzheimer's Association (US) *Fact Sheet: AN-1792*, http://www.alz. org/ResourceCenter/ByTopic/AN1792.htm [accessed December 5, 2002].

2   Check, E. 'Battle of the mind' *Nature*, Vol. 422, 2003, pp. 370–2.

3   Jorm, A. 'Prospects for the prevention of dementia' *Australasian Journal on Ageing*, Vol. 21, No. 1, 2001, pp. 9–13.

4   Alzheimer's Disease International Factsheet 9 *Risk Factors for Dementia*, Alzheimer's Disease International, London, October 2000.

5   Engelhart, M.J., Geerlings M.I., Ruitenberg, A. et al. 'Dietary intake of antioxidants and risk of Alzheimer disease' *JAMA*, Vol. 287, No. 24, 2002, pp. 3223–9.

6   Morris, M.C., Evans, D.A., Bienias, J.L. et al. 'Vitamin E and cognitive decline in older persons' *Archives of Neurology*, Vol. 59, No. 7, 2002, pp. 1125–32.

7   Foley, D.J. and White, L.R. 'Dietary intake of antioxidants and risk of Alzheimer's disease: Food for thought' *JAMA*, Vol. 287, No. 24, 2002, pp. 3261–3.

8   Ruitenberg, A., van Swieten, J.C., Witteman, J.C.M. et al. 'Alcohol consumption and risk of dementia: The Rotterdam Study' *The Lancet*, Vol. 359, No. 9303, January 26, 2002, pp. 281–6.

9   Truelsen, T., Thudium, D. and Grønbæk, M. 'Amount and type of alcohol and risk of dementia: The Copenhagen City heart study' *Neurology*, Vol. 59, 2002, pp. 1313–19.

10 Jorm, A. 'Prospects for the prevention of dementia' *Australasian Journal on Ageing*, Vol. 21, No. 1, 2001, pp. 9–13.

11 Snowdon, D. 'The Nun Study—frequently asked questions' http://www.mc.uky.edu/nunnet/faq.htm [accessed December 6, 2002].

12 Schofield, P. 'Alzheimer's disease and brain reserve' *Australasian Journal on Ageing*, Vol. 18, No. 1, February 1999, pp. 10–14.

13 Wilson, R.S., Mendes de Leon, C.F., Barnes, L.L. et al. 'Participation in cognitively stimulating activities and risk of incident Alzheimer disease' *JAMA*, Vol. 287, 2002, pp. 742–8.

14 Alzheimer's Disease Education and Referral Center, National Institute on Aging *Gingko Biloba Fact Sheet* http://www.alzheimers.org/pubs/gingko.html [accessed December 6, 2002].

15 Hogervorst, E., Ribeiro, H.M., Molyneux, A. et al. 'Plasma homocysteine levels, cerebrovascular risk factors, and cerebral white matter changes (leukoaraiosis) in patients with Alzheimer disease' *Archives of Neurology*, Vol. 59, No. 5, 2002, pp. 787–93.

16 Barberger-Gateau, P., Letenneur, L., Deschamps, V. et al. 'Fish, meat, and risk of dementia: Cohort study' *British Medical Journal*, Vol. 325, 2002, pp. 932–3.

17   Maia, L. and de Mendonca, A. 'Does caffeine intake protect from Alzheimer's disease?' *European Journal of Neurology*, Vol. 9, No. 4, 2002, pp. 377–82.

CHAPTER 3

1   Liddell, M.B., Lovestone, S. and Owen, M.J. 'Genetic risk of Alzheimer's disease: Advising relatives' *British Journal of Psychiatry*, Vol. 178, 2001, pp. 7–11.
2   ibid., pp 7–11.
3   Schmidt, R., Schmidt, H. and Fazekas, F. 'Vascular risk factors in dementia' *Journal of Neurology*, Vol. 247, 2000, pp. 81–7.
4   Kivipelto, M., Helkala, E.L., Laakso, M.P. et al. 'Midlife vascular risk factors and Alzheimer's disease in later life: Longitudinal, population based study' *British Medical Journal*, Vol. 322, No. 7300, 2001, pp. 1447–51.
5   Jorm, A. 'Prospects for the prevention of dementia' *Australasian Journal on Ageing*, Vol. 21, No. 1, 2001, pp. 9–13.
6   PROGRESS Collaborative Group 'Randomised trial of a perindopril-based blood pressure lowering regimen among 6105 individuals with previous stroke or transient ischaemic attack' *The Lancet*, Vol. 358, No. 9287, 2001, pp. 1033–41.
7   Almeida, O.P., Hulse, G.K., Lawrence, D. et al. 'Smoking as a risk factor for Alzheimer's disease: Contrasting evidence from a systematic review of case-control and cohort studies' *Addiction*, Vol. 97, No. 1, January 2002, pp. 15–28.
8   Stewart, R. and Liolitsa, D. 'Type 2 diabetes mellitus, cognitive impairment and dementia' *Diabetic Medicine*, Vol. 12, No. 2, 1999, pp. 93–112.
9   Newman, M.F., Kirchner, J.L., Phillips-Bute, B. et al. 'Longitudinal assessment of neurocognitive function after coronary-artery bypass surgery' *The New England Journal of Medicine*, Vol. 344, No. 6, 2001, pp. 395–402.
10 Kivipelto, M., Helkala, E.L., Laakso, M.P. et al. 'Midlife vascular risk factors and Alzheimer's disease in later life: Longitudinal, population based study' *British Medical Journal*, Vol. 322, No. 7300, 2001, pp. 1447–51.
11 Alzheimer's Association (US) *8th International Conference on Alzheimer's Disease and Related Disorders* http://www.alz.org/internationalconference/Pressreleases/PR_072302_C.htm [accessed December 6, 2002].
12 Rockwood, K., Kirkland, S., Hogan, D.B. et al. 'Use of lipid-lowering agents, indication bias, and the risk of dementia in community-dwelling elderly people' *Archives of Neurology*, Vol. 59, No. 2, 2002, pp. 223–7.

13   Alzheimer's Association (US) *8th International Conference on Alzheimer's Disease and Related Disorders* http://www.alz.org/internationalconference/Pressreleases/PR_072302_C.htm [accessed December 6, 2002].

14   Luchsinger, J.A., Tang, M-X., Shea, S. et al. 'Caloric intake and the risk of Alzheimer's disease' *Archives of Neurology*, Vol. 59, 2002, pp. 1258–63.

15   Gustafson, D., Rothenberg, E., Blennow, K., Steen, B., Skoog, I. 'An 18-year follow-up of overweight and risk of Alzheimer disease' *Archives Internal Medicine*, Vol. 163, 2003, pp. 1524–8.

16   LeBlanc, E.S., Janowsky, J., Chan, B.K.S. et al. 'Hormone replacement therapy and cognition: Systematic review and meta-analysis' *JAMA*, Vol. 285, 2001, pp. 1489–99; Zandi, P.P., Carlson, M.C., Plassman, B.L. et al. 'Hormone replacement therapy and incidence of Alzheimer's disease in older women: The Cache County Study' *JAMA*, Vol. 288, 2002, pp. 2123–9.

17   NIH News Release 'NHLBI stops trial of estrogen plus progestin due to increased breast cancer risk, lack of overall benefit' http://www.nhlbi.nih.gov/new/press/02-07-09.htm [accessed] December 7, 2002].

18   National Heart, Lung and Blood Institute *Facts about Post Menopausal Hormone Therapy* http://www.nhlbi.nih.gov/health/women/pht_facts.htm [accessed December 7, 2002].

19   NIA News: Alzheimer's disease research update *Free Testosterone Predictions Memory, Cognition in Older Men*, November 4, 2002 http://www.alzheimers.org/nianews/nianews48.html [accessed December 7, 2002].

20   't Veld, B.A., Ruitenberg, A., Hofman, A. et al. 'Nonsteroidal anti-inflammatory drugs and the risk of Alzheimer's disease' *New England Journal of Medicine*, Vol. 345, No. 21, 2001, pp. 1515–21.

21   Alzheimer's Association (US) *Fact Sheet: Anti-inflammatory Therapy* http://www.alz.org/ResourceCenter/ByTopic/antiinflammatory.htm [accessed December 7, 2002].

22   Helmer, C., Letenneur, L., Rouch, I. et al. 'Occupation during life and risk of dementia in French elderly community residents' *Journal of Neurology, Neurosurgery & Psychiatry*, Vol. 71, No. 3, 2001, pp. 303–9.

23   Jorm, A. 'Prospects for the prevention of dementia' *Australasian Journal of Ageing*, Vol. 21, 2001, pp. 9–13.

24   Tyas, S.L., Manfreda, J., Strain, L.A. et al. 'Risk factors for Alzheimer's disease: A population-based, longitudinal study in Manitoba, Canada' *International Journal of Epidemiology*, Vol. 30, No. 3, 2001, pp. 590–7.

25   Inouye, S.K., Bogardus, S.T. Jr, Baker, D.I. et al. 'The Hospital Elder Life Program: A model of care to prevent cognitive and functional decline in older hospitalised patients' *Journal of the American Geriatrics Society*, Vol. 48, No. 12, 2000, pp. 1697–706.

26   Petersen, R.C., Stevens, J.C., Ganguli, M. et al. 'Practice parameter: Early detection of dementia: Mild cognitive impairment (an evidence-based review)' *Neurology*, Vol. 56, 2001, pp. 1133–42.

27   Brodaty, H., Luscombe, G., Peisah, C. et al. 'A 25-year longitudinal comparison study of the outcome of depression' *Psychological Medicine*, Vol. 31, No. 8, 2001, pp. 1347–59.

28   National Institute on Aging *Alzheimer's Disease: Unravelling the Mystery* http://www.alzheimers.org/unravel.html [accessed December 7, 2002].

29   ibid.

30   ibid.

31   Chapman, M.R., Robinson, L.S., Pinkner, J.S. et al. 'Role of *Escherichia coli curli operons* in directing amyloid fiber formation' *Science*, Vol. 295, No. 5556, 2002, pp. 851–5.

CHAPTER 4

1   Brodaty, H. *Managing Alzheimer's Disease in Primary Care*, 2nd edn, Science Press, London, 1999.

2   International Psychogeriatric Association *Behavioral and Psychological Symptoms of Dementia (BPSD) Online Educational Pack* http://www.ipa-online.org/ipaonlinev3/ipaprograms/bpsd/ [accessed December 7, 2002].

3   Draper, B., Brodaty, H., Low, L-F. et al. 'Self destructive behaviours in nursing home residents' *Journal of the American Geriatrics Society*, Vol. 50, 2002, pp. 354–8.

CHAPTER 5

1   Lovestone, S. and McLoughlin, D.M. 'Protein aggregates and dementia: Is there a common toxicity?' *Journal of Neurology, Neurosurgery and Psychiatry*, Vol. 72, No. 2, 2002, pp. 152–61.

2   Tomlinson, B.E, Blessed, G. and Roth, M. 'Observations on the brains of demented old people' *Journal of Neurological Sciences*, Vol. 11, 1970, pp. 205–42.

3   National Institute on Aging *Progress Report on Alzheimer's Disease*, 2000 http://www.alzheimers.org/pubs/prog00.htm [accessed December 7, 2002].

4   Lovestone, S. 'Fleshing out the amyloid cascade hypothesis: The molecular biology of Alzheimer's disease' *Dialogues in Clinical Neuroscience*, Vol. 2, No. 2, 2000, pp. 101–10.

5   National Institute on Aging *Progress Report on Alzheimer's Disease*, 2000 http://www.alzheimers.org/pubs/prog00.htm [accessed December 7, 2002].

6   Masters, C. 'Genetic insights into the pathogenesis of Alzheimer's disease' *The Master Class in Alzheimer's Disease*, May 2002, Pfizer Neuroscience, Sydney, pp. 2–3.

7   National Institute on Aging. *Progress Report on Alzheimer's Disease*, 2000   http://www.alzheimers.org/pubs/prog00.htm   [accessed December 7, 2002].

8   ibid.

9   Gustafson, L. 'Historical overview' in E. Chiu, L. Gustafson, D. Ames and M.F. Folstein (eds) *Cerebrovascular Disease and Dementia*, Martin Dunitz Ltd, London, 2000, pp. 3–14.

10   Brun, A. 'The neuropathology of vascular dementia' in E. Chiu et al. (eds) *Cerebrovascular Disease and Dementia*, pp. 69–76.

11   Erkinjuntti, T. 'Classification and criteria' in E. Chiu et al. (eds) *Cerebrovascular Disease and Dementia*, pp. 99–113.

12   McKeith, I.G., Galasko, D., Kosaka, K. et al. 'Consensus guidelines for the clinical and pathologic diagnosis of dementia with Lewy bodies (DLB): Report of the consortium on DLB international workshop' *Neurology*, Vol. 47, 1996, pp. 1113–24.

13   ibid.

14   Lovestone, S. and McLoughlin, D.M. 'Protein aggregates and dementia: Is there a common toxicity?' *Journal of Neurology, Neurosurgery and Psychiatry*, Vol. 72, No. 2, 2002, pp. 152–61.

15   Neary, D., Snowden, J.S., Gustafson, L. et al. 'Frontotemporal lobar degeneration: A consensus on clinical diagnostic criteria' *Neurology*, Vol. 51, 1998, pp. 1546–54; Alzheimer's Association (US) Resource Center *Pick's Disease and Other Frontotemporal Dementias*, http://www.alz.org/ResourceCenter/ByTopic/RelatedDisorders. htm#frontotemporal [accessed December 7, 2002].

16   Lovestone, S. and McLoughlin, D.M. 'Protein aggregates and dementia', pp. 152–61.

17   ibid.

18   ibid.

19   National Institute on Aging *Progress Report on Alzheimer's Disease*, 2000   http://www.alzheimers.org/pubs/prog00.htm   [accessed December 7, 2002].

20   Draper, B. 'Potentially reversible dementia: A review' *Australian and New Zealand Journal of Psychiatry*, Vol. 25, 1991, pp. 506–18.

21   Welch, K. and Morse, A. 'The clinical profile of end-stage AIDS in the era of highly active antiretroviral therapy' *AIDS Patient Care & Stds*, Vol. 16, No. 2, 2002, pp. 75–81; Sacktor, N., McDermott, M.P., Marder, K. et al. 'HIV-associated cognitive impairment before and after the advent of combination therapy' *Journal of Neurovirology*, Vol. 8, No. 2, 2002, pp. 136–42; Dore, G.J., Correll, P.K., Li, Y. et al. 'Changes to AIDS dementia complex in the era of highly active antiretroviral therapy' *AIDS*, Vol. 13, No. 10, 1999, pp. 1249–53.

CHAPTER 6

1   Reisberg, B., Burns, A., Brodaty, H. et al. 'Diagnosis of Alzheimer's disease' *International Psychogeriatrics*, Vol. 9, Suppl. 1, 1997, pp. 11–38.

2   Brodaty, H., Pond, D., Kemp, N.M. et al. 'The GPCOG: A new
     screening test for dementia designed for general practice' *Journal of
     the American Geriatrics Society*, Vol. 50, 2002, pp. 530–4.
3   Sunderland, T. and Draper, B. 'Depression and dementia' in S. Findlay
     (ed) *Essentials of Dementia, Part Two*, Science Press, London, 2001.
4   Kiloh, L. 'Pseudo-dementia' *Acta Psychiatrica Scandinavica*, Vol. 37,
     1961, pp. 336–51.
5   Draper, B. 'Potentially reversible dementia: A review' *Australian and
     New Zealand Journal of Psychiatry*, Vol. 25, 1991, pp. 506–18.
6   Petersen, R.C., Stevens, J.C., Ganguli, M. et al. 'Practice para-
     meter: Early detection of dementia: Mild cognitive impairment
     (an evidence-based review)' *Neurology*, Vol. 56, 2001, pp. 1133–42.
7   Alzheimer's Association Help Sheet *Diagnosis: Informing the Person with
     Dementia*, http://www.alzvic.asn.au/ad17.htm [accessed December 8,
     2002].
8   Doody, R.S., Stevens, J.C., Beck, C. et al. 'Practice parameter:
     Management of dementia (an evidence-based review)' *Neurology*,
     Vol. 56, 2001, pp. 1154–66.

CHAPTER 7

1   Brodaty, H., Ames, D., Boundy, K.L. et al. 'Pharmacological treat-
     ment of cognitive deficits in Alzheimer's disease' *Medical Journal of
     Australia*, Vol. 175, 2001, pp. 324–9.
2   *MIMS Australia*, Vol. 39, No. 4, 2002, pp. 103–5.
3   National Institute on Aging *Gingko Biloba Fact Sheet* http://www.
     alzheimers.org/pubs/gingko.html [accessed December 10, 2002].
4   Brodaty, H., Ames, D., Boundy, K.L. et al. 'Pharmacological treat-
     ment of cognitive deficits in Alzheimer's disease' pp. 324–9.
5   ibid.
6   Alzheimer's Association (US) *Fact Sheet: Memantine* http://
     www.alz.org/ResourceCenter/ByTopic/memantine.htm [accessed
     December 10, 2002].
7   Alzheimer's Association (US) *Alternative Treatments* http://www.
     alz.org/PhysCare/Treating/treatments.htm [accessed December 10,
     2002].
8   International Psychogeriatric Association *Behavioral and
     Psychological Symptoms of Dementia (BPSD) Online Educational Pack*
     http://www.ipa-online.org/ipaonlinev3/ipaprograms/bpsd/
     [accessed December 7, 2002]; Brodaty, H. *Managing Alzheimer's
     Disease in Primary Care*, 2nd edn, Science Press, London, 1999.
9   Draper, B., Brodaty, H., Low, L.-F. et al. 'Use of psychotropics in
     Sydney nursing homes: Associations with psychosis, depression and
     behavioural disturbances' *International Psychogeriatrics*, Vol. 13,
     2001, pp. 107–20.
10   Sunderland, T. and Draper, B. 'Depression and dementia' in S. Findlay
     (ed.) *Essentials of Dementia, Part Two*, Science Press, London, 2001.

CHAPTER 8

1   Kitwood, T. 'Person and process in dementia' *International Journal of Geriatric Psychiatry*, Vol. 8, 1993, pp. 541–5; Woods, R.T. 'Discovering the person with Alzheimer's disease: Cognitive, emotional and behavioural aspects' *Aging & Mental Health*, Vol. 5, Suppl. 1, 2001, S7–S16.

2   Gatz, M., Fiske, A., Fox, L.S. et al. 'Empirically validated psychological treatments for older adults' *Journal of Mental Health and Aging*, Vol. 4, No. 1, 1998, p. 34.

3   Jones, G. 'A review of Feil's validation method for communicating with and caring for dementia sufferers' *Current Opinion in Psychiatry*, Vol. 10, No. 4, 1997, pp. 326–32.

4   Neill, M. and Briggs, M. 'Validation therapy for dementia' *Cochrane Database of Systematic Reviews*, Issue 2, 2002.

5   Gatz, M., Fiske, A., Fox, L.S. et al. 'Empirically validated psychological treatments for older adults' *Journal of Mental Health and Aging*, Vol. 4, No. 1, 1998, p. 35.

6   ibid., pp. 35–6.

7   Opie, J., Rosewarne, R., O'Connor, D.W. 'The efficacy of psychosocial approaches to behaviour disorders in dementia: A systematic literature review' *Australian and New Zealand Journal of Psychiatry*, Vol. 33, 1999, pp. 789–99.

8   ibid.

9   ibid; Gassib-Spain, L., Stewart, A., Tranter, S. et al. *Complementary Therapies and Nursing Practice*, South East Health, Dolls Point, 2001.

10 Opie, J., Rosewarne, R., O'Connor, D.W. 'The efficacy of psychosocial approaches to behaviour disorders in dementia: A systematic literature review' *Australian and New Zealand Journal of Psychiatry*, Vol. 33, 1999, pp. 789–99.

11 Doyle, C., Zapparoni, T., O'Connor, D. et al. 'Efficacy of psychosocial treatments for noisemaking in severe dementia' *International Psychogeriatrics*, Vol. 9, No. 4, 1997, pp. 405–22; Bird, M., Alexopoulos, P. and Adamowicz, J. 'Success and failure in five case studies: Use of cued recall to ameliorate behaviour problems in senile dementia' *International Journal of Geriatric Psychiatry*, Vol. 10, 1995, pp. 305–11.

12 Draper, B., Turner, J., McMinn, B. et al. 'Treatment outcomes of nursing home residents with vocally disruptive behaviour' *Australasian Journal on Ageing*, Vol. 22, No. 2, 2003, pp. 81–5.

13 Zisselman, M.H., Rovner, B.W., Shmuely, Y. et al. 'A pet therapy intervention with geriatric psychiatry inpatients' *The American Journal of Occupational Therapy*, Vol. 50, No. 1, 1996, pp. 47–51.

14 Opie, J., Rosewarne, R., O'Connor, D.W. 'The efficacy of psychosocial approaches to behaviour disorders in dementia: A systematic

literature review' *Australian and New Zealand Journal of Psychiatry*, Vol. 33, 1999, pp. 789–99.

15   Dowling, Z., Baker, R., Wareing, L.A. et al. 'Lights, sound and special effects?' *Journal of Dementia Care*, Vol. 5, No. 1, 1997, pp. 16–18.

16   Retsas, A. 'Use of physical restraints in South Australia's nursing homes' *Australian Journal on Ageing*, Vol. 16, 1997, pp. 169–73.

CHAPTER 9

1   Mace, N. and Rabins, P. *The 36-Hour Day: A Family Guide to Caring for Persons with Alzheimer's Disease, Related Dementing Illnesses, and Memory Loss in Later Life*, 3rd edn; Johns Hopkins University Press, Baltimore, 1999.

2   Liddell, M.B., Lovestone, S. and Owen, M.J. 'Genetic risk of Alzheimer's disease: Advising relatives' *British Journal of Psychiatry*, Vol. 178, 2001, pp. 7–11.

3   West, L. 'My dad' *Global Perspective*, Vol. 11, No. 2, July 2001, p. 3.

4   Alzheimer's Association Australia *Young People and Dementia* http://www.alzvic.asn.au/hsyoungpeople.htm [accessed December 13, 2002].

5   Australian Institute of Health and Welfare *Residential Aged Care in Australia 2000–01: A Statistical Overview* http://www.aihw.gov.au/publications/age/racsa00-01/index.html [accessed December 13, 2002].

6   Cooney, C. and Howard, R. 'Abuse of patients with dementia by carers—out of sight but not out of mind' *International Journal of Geriatric Psychiatry*, Vol. 10, 1995, pp. 735–41; Sadler, P., Kurrle, S., Cameron, I. 'Dementia and elder abuse' *Australasian Journal on Ageing*, Vol. 14, No. 1, 1995, pp. 36–40.

7   Franzen, J. 'Into the abyss' *Good Weekend*, May 11, 2002, pp. 45–54.

8   Morris, R.G., Woods, R.T., Davies, K.S. et al. 'Gender differences in carers of dementia sufferers' *British Journal of Psychiatry*, Vol. 158, Suppl. 10, 1991, pp. 69–74.

9   Gutmann, D. 'Psychological development and pathology in later adulthood' in R. Nemiroff and C. Colarusso (eds) *New Dimensions in Adult Development*, Basic Books, New York, 1990, pp. 170–84.

10   Brodaty, H., Gresham, M. and Luscombe, G. 'The Prince Henry Hospital dementia caregivers training programme' *International Journal of Geriatric Psychiatry*, Vol. 12, No. 2, 1997, pp. 183–92.

CHAPTER 10

1   Howe, A.L. 'From states of confusion to a National Action Plan for Dementia Care: The development of policies for dementia care in Australia' *International Journal of Geriatric Psychiatry*, Vol. 12, No. 2, 1997, pp. 165–72.

2   Department of Community Services and Health *Nursing Homes and Hostels Review*, Australian Government Publishing Service, Canberra, 1986.
3   ibid., p. 3.
4   Howe, A.L. 'From states of confusion to a National Action Plan for Dementia Care: The development of policies for dementia care in Australia' *International Journal of Geriatric Psychiatry*, Vol. 12, No. 2, 1997, pp. 165–72.
5   Aged and Community Services Australia Community Care Reform Project Community Care Reference Group *A Vision for Community Care: A Discussion Paper, August 2002* http://agedcare.org.au/projects/communitycare/community_care_vision1308.pdf [accessed December 14, 2002].
6   Australian Department of Health and Ageing *Aged Care Assessment Teams* http://www.health.gov.au/acc/acat/assess.htm [accessed December 14, 2002].
7   Australian Department of Health and Ageing *Aged Care Assessment Program Operational Guidelines* http://www.health.gov.au/acc/acat/acapopgu.htm [accessed December 14, 2002].
8   ibid.
9   ibid.
10 Australian Department of Health and Ageing *Home and Community Care (HACC) Program* http://www.health.gov.au/acc/hacc/abthacc.htm [accessed December 14, 2002].
11 Australian Department of Health and Ageing *Guidelines for the Home and Community Care Program National Service Standards* http://www.health.gov.au/acc/hacc/girindex.htm [accessed December 14, 2002].
12 Australian Department of Health and Ageing *Commonwealth Carer Resource Centres* http://www.health.gov.au/acc/carers/resocent.htm [accessed December 14, 2002].
13 Australian Department of Health and Ageing *Respite Care and Other Services for Carers* http://www.health.gov.au/acc/publicat/qcoa/04info.htm [accessed December 14, 2002].
14 Gray, L. *Two Year Review of Aged Care Reforms*, Department of Health and Aged Care, Canberra, 2001, p. 37.
15 Australian Department of Health and Ageing *Respite Care and Other Services for Carers* http://www.health.gov.au/acc/publicat/qcoa/04info.htm [accessed December 14, 2002].
16 Centrelink *Carer Allowance* http://www.centrelink.gov.au/internet/internet.nsf/payments/carer_allow_adult.htm [accessed December 14, 2002].
17 Centrelink *Carer Payment* http://www.centrelink.gov.au/internet/internet.nsf/payments/carer.htm [accessed December 14, 2002].
18 Australian Department of Health and Ageing *Community Aged Care*

Packages (CACPs) http://www.health.gov.au/acc/commcare/cacp.
htm [accessed December 14, 2002].

19 Australian Institute of Health and Welfare *Community Aged Care Packages in Australia, 2000–01, A Statistical Overview* http://www.aihw.gov.au/publications/age/cacpa00-01/cacpa00-01.pdf [accessed December 14, 2002].

20 Challis, D., von Abendorff, R., Brown, P. et al. 'Care management, dementia care and specialist mental health services: An evaluation' *International Journal of Geriatric Psychiatry*, Vol. 17, 2002, pp. 315–25.

21 Australian Department of Health and Ageing *Extended Aged Care at Home Packages Pilot* http://www.health.gov.au/acc/commcare/comcprov/eachdex.htm [accessed December 14, 2002].

22 Aged and Community Services Australia Community Care Reform Project Community Care Reference Group *A Vision for Community Care: A Discussion Paper, August 2002* http://agedcare.org.au/projects/communitycare/community_care_vision1308.pdf, p. 2, [accessed December 14, 2002].

CHAPTER 11

1 Australian Department of Health and Ageing *Aged Care Assessment Program Operational Guidelines* http://www.health.gov.au/acc/acat/acapopgu.htm [accessed December 14, 2002].

2 Australian Department of Health and Ageing *Residential Care Manual* http://www.health.gov.au/acc/manuals/rcm/contents/1intro.htm [accessed December 14, 2002].

3 Draper, B., Snowdon, J., Meares, S. et al. 'Case-controlled study of nursing home residents referred for treatment of vocally disruptive behavior' *International Psychogeriatrics*, Vol. 12, 2000, pp. 333–44.

4 Morley, J.E. and Flaherty, J.H. 'Putting the "home" back in nursing home' *Journal of Gerontology: Medical Sciences*, Vol. 57A, No. 7, 2002, M419–21; Brawley, E.C. 'Environmental design for Alzheimer's disease: A quality of life issue' *Ageing & Mental Health*, Vol. 5, Suppl. 1, 2001, S79–83; Hoskins, G. and Marshall, M. 'Expect more: Making a place for people with dementia' in R. Jacoby and C. Oppenheimer (eds) *Psychiatry in the Elderly*, 3rd edn, Oxford University Press, Oxford, 2002, pp. 460–83.

5 Gray, L. *Two Year Review of Aged Care Reforms*, Department of Health and Aged Care, Canberra, 2001, pp. 5–6.

6 Australian Institute of Health and Welfare 'Dementia and older Australians' in *Older Australia at a Glance (2nd edn), 1999* http://www.aihw.gov.au/publications/welfare/oag/oag-c09.html [accessed December 14, 2002].

7 ibid.

8 ibid.

9   Sloane, P.D., Lindeman, D.A., Phillips, C. et al. 'Evaluating Alzheimer's special care units: Reviewing the evidence and identifying potential sources of study bias' *The Gerontologist*, Vol. 35, No. 1, 1995, pp. 103–11.

10   Australian Department of Health and Ageing *Residential Care Manual* http://www.health.gov.au/acc/manuals/rcm/contents/1intro.htm [accessed December 14, 2002].

11   Andrews, K. *New Funding Scheme to Relieve Nurse's Paperwork, May 9, 2002* http://www.health.gov.au/mediarel/yr2002/ka/ka02029.htm [accessed December 14, 2002].

12   Australian Department of Health and Ageing *Financial Information* http://www.health.gov.au/acc/finance/fininfo.htm [accessed December 14, 2002].

13   Gray, L. *Two Year Review of Aged Care Reforms*, Department of Health and Aged Care, Canberra, 2001, pp. 77–117.

14   Australian Department of Health and Ageing *Sanctions Update* http://www.health.gov.au/acc/rescare/sanction.htm [accessed December 14, 2002].

15   Gray, L. 'Beyond the two year review: The new generation of issues in aged care' *Australasian Journal on Ageing*, Vol. 20, No. 3, 2001, pp. 123–6.

CHAPTER 12

1   Perkins, C.J. 'Ethical issues in geriatric psychiatry liaison' in P. Melding and B. Draper (eds) *Geriatric Consultation Liaison Psychiatry*, Oxford University Press, Oxford, 2001, pp. 337–9.

2   NSW Young Lawyers *Older People and the Law*, Law Society of New South Wales, Sydney, 2002.

3   Molloy, D.W., Darzins, P., Strang, D. *Capacity to Decide*, New Grange Press, Troy, Ontario, 1999, pp. 21–30.

4   New South Wales Consolidated Acts *Guardianship Act 1987* http://www.austlii.edu.au/au/legis/nsw/consol_act/ga1987136/ [accessed December 15, 2002].

5   Hertogh, C.M.P.M. and Ribbe, M.W. 'Ethical aspects of medical decision-making in demented patients: A report from the Netherlands' *Alzheimer's Disease and Associated Disorders*, Vol. 10, No. 1, 1996, pp. 11–19.

6   NSW Young Lawyers *Older People and the Law*, Law Society of New South Wales, Sydney, 2002.

7   New South Wales Consolidated Acts *Guardianship Act 1987* http://www.austlii.edu.au/au/legis/nsw/consol_act/ga1987136/ [accessed December 15, 2002].

8   ibid.

9   Dubinsky, R.M., Stein, A.C., Lyons, K. 'Practice parameter: Risk of driving and Alzheimer's disease (an evidence based review). Report

of the Quality Standards Subcommittee of the American Academy of Neurology' *Neurology*, Vol. 54, 2000, pp. 2205–11.

10   Austroads Working Party *Assessing Fitness to Drive*, Austroads, Sydney, 2001, p. 43.

11   Angley, P. 'Driving and dementia: A background paper' *Alzheimer's Association Victoria*, June 2001. http://www.alzheimers.org.au/drivingaavpaper.pdf [accessed December 15, 2002, pp. 13–14].

12   Dubinsky, R.M., Stein, A.C., Lyons, K. 'Practice parameter' pp. 2205–11.

13   Angley, P. 'Driving and dementia' http://www.alzheimers.org.au/drivingaavpaper.pdf [accessed December 15, 2002, pp. 7–8].

14   Austroads Working Party *Assessing Fitness to Drive*, Austroads, Sydney, 2001, p. 43.

15   Berghmans, R.L.P. and Ter Meulen, R.H.J. 'Ethical issues in research with dementia patients' *International Journal of Geriatric Psychiatry*, Vol. 10, 1995, pp. 647–51; Appelbaum, P.S. 'Involving decisionally impaired subjects in research' *American Journal of Geriatric Psychiatry*, Vol. 10, No. 2, 2002, pp. 120–4.

16   Hughes, J.C. 'Ethics and the anti-dementia drugs' *International Journal of Geriatric Psychiatry*, Vol. 15, 2000, pp. 538–43.

17   Hughes, J.C. and Louw, S.J. 'Electronic tagging of people with dementia who wander' *British Medical Journal*, Vol. 325, No. 7369, 2002, p. 847.

18   Lambourne, P. and Lambourne, A. 'Do not resuscitate policies: What do staff and relatives want for patients with severe dementia?' *International Journal of Geriatric Psychiatry*, Vol. 16, 2001, pp. 1107–9.

19   Cartwright, C.M. and Steinberg, M.A. 'PEG feeding, dementia and the need for policies and guidelines' *Australasian Journal on Ageing*, Vol. 19, No. 3, 2000, pp. 106–7; Alzheimer's Association (US) *Assisted Oral Feeding and Tube Feeding* http://www.alz.org/ResourceCenter/FactSheets/FSOralfeeding.pdf [accessed December 15, 2002].

CHAPTER 13

1   The Ronald and Nancy Reagan Research Institute of the Alzheimer's Association and the National Institute on Aging Working Group 'Consensus Report of the Working Group on: Molecular and biochemical markers of Alzheimer's disease' *Neurobiology of Aging*, Vol. 19, No. 2, 1998, pp. 109–16.

2   Riemenschneider, M., Lautenschlager, N., Wagenpfeil, S. et al. 'Cerebrospinal fluid tau and beta-amyloid 42 proteins identify Alzheimer Disease in subjects with mild cognitive impairment' *Archives of Neurology*, Vol. 59, No. 11, 2002, pp. 1729–34.

3   Toga, A.W. and Thompson, P.M. 'New approaches in brain

morphometry' *American Journal of Geriatric Psychiatry*, Vol. 10, No. 1, 2002, pp. 13–23.

4 Alexander, G.E., Chen, K., Pietrini, P. et al. 'Longitudinal PET evaluation of cerebral metabolic decline in dementia: A potential outcome measure in Alzheimer's disease treatment studies' *American Journal of Psychiatry*, Vol. 159, 2002, pp. 738–45.

5 Shoghi-Jadid, K., Small, G.W., Agdeppa, E.D. et al. 'Localization of neurofibrillary tangles and beta-amyloid plaques in the brains of living patients with Alzheimer's disease' *American Journal of Geriatric Psychiatry*, Vol. 10, 2002, pp. 24–35.

6 Bookheimer, S.Y., Strojwas, M.H., Cohen, M.S. et al. 'Patterns of brain activation in people at risk for Alzheimer's disease' *The New England Journal of Medicine*, Vol. 343, No. 7, 2000, pp. 450–6.

7 CogState http://www.cogstate.com/cogstate/index.html [accessed December 15, 2002].

8 Alzheimer's Disease Clinical Trials Database *A Phase I Study of ex vivo Nerve Growth Factor Gene Therapy for Alzheimer's Disease* http://www.alzheimers.org/dbtw-wpd/exec/dbtwpcgi.exe?BU= http://www.alzheimers.org/aztrials/basicsearch.html&QB0=AND &QF0=Study_ID&QI0=IA0029&TN=trials&DF=Full+Records& RF=Full+Records&DL=1&RL=1&NP=1&AC=QBE_QUERY [accessed December 15, 2002].

9 Galvin, K.A. and Jones, D.G. 'Adult human neural stem cells for cell-replacement therapies in the central nervous system' *Medical Journal of Australia*, Vol. 177, No. 6, 2002, pp. 316–18.

10 Alzheimer's Association (US) *Resource Center: Fact Sheets* http://www.alz.org/ResourceCenter/ByType/FactSheets.htm [accessed December 15, 2002].

INDEX

DATE DUE